Expressing Your Milk

Excerpt from Working and Breastfeeding Made Simple

Nancy Mohrbacher, IBCLC, FILCA

Praeclarus Press, LLC

www.PraeclarusPress.com

Praeclarus Press, LLC
2504 Sweetgum Lane
Amarillo, Texas 79124 USA
806-367-9950
www.PraeclarusPress.com

DISCLAIMER

The information contained in this publication is advisory only and is not intended to replace sound clinical judgment or individualized patient care. The author disclaims all warranties, whether expressed or implied, including any warranty as the quality, accuracy, safety, or suitability of this information for any particular purpose.

ISBN: 978-1-939807-46-5
©2016 Nancy Mohrbacher. All rights reserved.

Cover Design: Ken Tackett
Acquisition & Development: Kathleen Kendall-Tackett
Copy Editing: Chris Tackett
Layout & Design: Nelly Murariu
Operations: Scott Sherwood

Table of Contents

1

Intro

If you're reading this, chances are you are planning to pump and provide your milk for your baby when your baby cannot directly feed from your breasts. Why do you need this book? First, you'll find tips and insights that can simplify your life and make the process less confusing. Second, despite the information available, without some inside knowledge, you're unlikely to meet your breastfeeding goals. I chose this book's content to help you avoid the experience of women who did not reach their breastfeeding goals.

Why Breastfeeding Matters

Most mothers know that babies who are not breastfed are at greater risk for many health problems. But only recently have we begun to understand the risk to mothers when breastfeeding is cut short. Breastfeeding is not just important to your baby. It's also important to you.

Breastfeeding and You

Breastfeeding is a key women's health issue. A growing body of research has linked a lack of breastfeeding and early weaning to the number one killer of women, heart disease, as well as breast and ovarian cancers, metabolic syndrome, type 2 diabetes, and many other serious health problems. Breastfeeding even affects your response to stress (helping you cope with it better), your resistance to illness (boosting it), and how well and how long you sleep (longer and deeper).

For years, people assumed that breastfeeding was draining to mothers. While fatigue is a normal part of life for all new parents, it turns out this assumption was dead wrong. Your body adapts to lactation by reducing the energy required to make milk, which also improves your other body functions. Scientists think that milk-making actually "primes" or "resets" your metabolism after birth to boost your metabolic efficiency (Stuebe & Rich-Edwards, 2009). Lactation improves digestion and increases absorption of nutrients (Hammond, 1997). It increases your sensitivity to the hormone insulin in the short and long term. For every year you breastfeed, over the next 15 years, your risk of developing type 2 diabetes decreases by about 15% (Stuebe, Rich-Edwards, Willett, Manson, & Michels, 2005).

Breastfeeding and Your Baby

Thousands of studies have reported on the health drawbacks when babies are not breastfed. The American Academy of Pediatrics 2012 Policy Statement recommends exclusive breastfeeding for the first six months and a minimum of one year of total breastfeeding (AAP, 2012). Babies who are *not breastfed* are at increased risk of these health problems.

- 72% increased risk of lower respiratory infections
- 63% increased risk of upper respiratory infections
- 50% increased risk of ear infections
- 40% increased risk of asthma
- 42% increased risk of allergic rashes
- 64% increased risk of digestive tract infections
- 30% increased risk of type 1 diabetes
- 36% increased risk of Sudden Infant Death Syndrome

But a healthier first year is not the end of the story. One compelling reason that one year of breastfeeding is recommended is that these health differences are not restricted to infancy. Babies who do not breastfeed or who wean early are more likely to develop the following conditions as they mature: obesity, diabetes, inflammatory bowel diseases, celiac disease, and childhood leukemia and lymphoma. For an overview of why breastfeeding matters from a health standpoint to both you and your baby, see the 2010 article "The Risks and Benefits of Infant Feeding Practices for Women and Their Children" (Stuebe & Schwarz, 2010): *http://www.ncbi.nlm.nih.gov/pmc/articles/PMC2812877/ pdf/RIOG002004_0222.pdf*.

In order to make a truly informed decisions, parents need to know how breastfeeding impacts lifelong health. When it comes to breastfeeding, knowledge is definitely power. Knowing what's at stake may help you get through the rough spots that many breastfeeding mothers experience.

For many women, though, the importance of breastfeeding to health isn't even on their radar. Breastfeeding's main appeal is that it increases the connection between mother and baby. When you and your baby are regularly apart, your emotional connection with your baby looms large, as Marge describes.

I loved that this was something only I could do for my baby. I was worried he would think his nanny was his mom, but everyone reassured me children always know who the mom is—from the intensity of the relationship and connection. Still, the breastfeeding and providing all his milk made me feel connected, a 24/7 mom.

—*Marge G., Ohio, USA*

How can you make breastfeeding—and the close connection that it fosters—a reality? That's what this book is about.

Let Me Be Your Guide

My love for breastfeeding began when I breastfed my own three sons, who are now grown. I started working with mothers as a volunteer in 1982. After I became board-certified, for 10 years, I ran a large private lactation practice in the Chicago area, where I worked one-on-one with thousands of families. I also worked for eight years as a lactation consultant for a major breast pump company, educating health care providers and answering mothers' questions about milk supply and how to make the most of a breast pump. I wrote breastfeeding books used worldwide by parents and professionals, which has kept me current in the lactation research. When I began writing this book, I worked in a corporate lactation program, where I talked daily to women who were pregnant, on maternity leave, and who had returned to work. As you can probably tell, I have a passion for helping breastfeeding mothers. I'd love to share what I've learned with you.

In this book, I've included the key ingredients that make breastfeeding work. It's not complicated. In fact, much of it is very simple. But without this information, working and breastfeeding may be more difficult or more worrisome than it needs to be. These pages include the latest on many of the burning issues you may face: milk production, maternity leave, pumping, flexible job options, childcare, milk storage and handling, work-life balance, and much, much more.

But before we get into these specifics, let me circle back to the sobering figures I mentioned in the beginning on how many women wean earlier than intended. I'd like to explain some of the dynamics that affect these numbers.

The Challenges in Brief

Why is breastfeeding so challenging for so many mothers? One reason is that many mothers and babies don't get the help they need from the institutions that touch their lives. For example, the U.S. Centers for Disease Control and Prevention report that after birth, one in every four U.S. newborns is supplemented in the hospital with infant formula (Centers for Disease Control and Prevention, 2012). Giving newborns formula unnecessarily is a common first step to milk-production problems. Science tells us that worry about milk production is the number one reason women wean before they'd planned. Because many health professionals receive no breastfeeding training, they often give mothers conflicting advice while they are still in the hospital. And some of this advice undermines mothers' best efforts to breastfeed.

After mother and baby arrive home, if breastfeeding problems develop, skilled help is not always affordable or easy to find. When maternity leave ends, many women find their workplaces lack the support they need to continue breastfeeding.

At this writing, a recently upheld U.S. health care law, the Affordable Care Act, is now in place. According to this law, the costs of breastfeeding supplies and services for new mothers should be covered by health insurance. How this law's provisions will translate into reality is still unclear. As always, the devil is in the details.

Weaning earlier than intended, however, is not always the result of health care or worksite challenges. It has a much more personal side. Another major reason so many women stop nursing before they had planned is that they are confused about what's normal and how breastfeeding works (DaMota, Banuelos, Goldbronn, Vera-Beccera, & Heinig, 2012). My hope is that this book will provide an antidote to this confusion so that you can experience the empowerment that comes from reaching your breastfeeding goals.

Maternity Leave

The length of your maternity leave is a big piece of this puzzle. Paid maternity leave is available in almost every country, but the details vary from place to place. In Sweden, for example, one year of paid maternity leave is standard, and fathers also have six months of paid leave. In Canada, depending on how long a mother has been at her job and how many hours per week she works, she may be eligible for 15 weeks of paid leave at full salary with an option to take up to 52 weeks at partial salary and her job guaranteed. Yet not all Canadian mothers take advantage of this.

In the U.K., mothers receive 90% of their weekly salary for the first six weeks after birth and the option of up to 52 weeks maternity leave. After the first six weeks, they can stay home at a flat rate for the next 33 weeks, and the last 13 weeks are unpaid. In Australia, 12 months unpaid leave is guaranteed, and the Australian government pays employers (who pass this on to mothers) up to 18 weeks of pay at the national minimum wage, in addition to whatever job benefits mothers receive. But even where paid maternity leave is available, some women do not take advantage of it.

In the United States, under the Family and Medical Leave Act, 12 weeks of unpaid leave is the law of the land, but that's only for those working full time in companies with more than 50 employees. For many American women, any maternity leave—paid or unpaid—is just a dream. But because maternity leave in the U.S. is tied to job benefits, some have more leeway than others. Women employed at the upper levels of large corporations may receive six months or more of paid leave, while women in low-income jobs may have no leave at all and be forced by money pressures to return to work within weeks—or even days—after giving birth.

How This Book Can Help

No matter where you live or what kind of work you do, knowing how the length of your maternity leave affects your back-to-work planning may give you a useful perspective. That's what the first chapter is about. Even if you have no say in your maternity leave, these insights will give you a better idea of what to expect. Hopefully, having this big picture will help you put the sometimes-confusing details into place.

My fondest hope is that this book will help you achieve your personal goals. Especially during the early weeks, expressing your milk can sometimes feel like a marathon. But like a marathon, crossing the finish line can be a real peak experience. And like the effort that goes into preparing for a race, the more you put into itp, the more you can relish the elation that comes with such an outstanding achievement. Between now and then, I'll be cheering you on.

Nancy Mohrbacher
Arlington Heights, IL USA

2

Breast Pump Choice and Fit

If you've never used a breast pump, the whole idea of pumping your milk may seem strange and even off-putting. If you plan to use a pump, learning a little about it may help you feel more at ease. But before getting into these specifics, know up front that like breastfeeding, pumping is not supposed to hurt. A key part of comfortable pumping is choosing a pump that's right for your situation and one that fits you well, which this chapter explains in more detail.

Your Situation and Pump Choice

If you plan to use a breast pump, the first step is deciding which type of pump to get. It's easy to feel confused by the large array of breast pumps online and on store shelves. Knowing which type of pump is better suited to which situations may narrow your choices and make this process easier. How often you plan to pump, and your reason for pumping, can help you decide on the best pump for you. Below are some common reasons why women need a pump.

Your Newborn Isn't Breastfeeding or Your Supply Needs a Boost

The recommended pumps in these situations are those used in hospitals. You will probably rent this type of pump, and the pump motor is shared. Each mother buys her own milk collection kit (the parts that come into contact with the milk), so one mother's milk never touches another's. A double milk-collection kit lets you pump both breasts at the same time (double pumping), which takes half the time of pumping one breast at a time (single pumping). These pumps (Figure 1) are larger and heavier than those purchased for home or office use, because they are made to be durable enough to be used by many women. See the Resources section for website URLs of the three major brands of rental pumps: Ameda, Hygeia, and Medela. You can find the closest pump rental business near you online.

Some of these pumps provide slightly stronger suction than the pumps you can buy, but that's not why they're recommended. Most provide a smoother feel, and more suction and speed settings. These differences make them the best choice when a baby is not nursing at all or when milk production needs a boost.

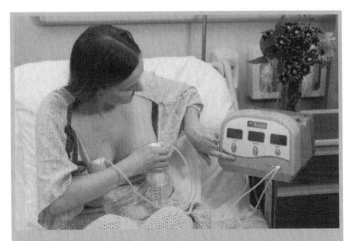

Figure 1. This mother, who is pumping in the hospital for a premature baby, uses one arm to double pump so she has a hand free to adjust her rental pump's controls. ©2014 Ameda, Inc. Used with permission.

You're Pumping Daily

If you'll be pumping once a day or more often, consider buying a double-electric breast pump with a motor warranty of at least one year. (Those with shorter warranties may not be durable enough to meet your needs.) These pumps are sometimes called "professional grade," and are not recommended for sharing, because their motors are not heavy-duty enough to work properly after multiple users (see Figure 2). Some brands are not safe to share for hygiene reasons (see later section on used breast pumps).

These pumps come with a double milk-collection kit so pumping takes half the time of single pumping. Whatever your work setting, if you'll be doing a lot of pumping, the total time spent is important. These pumps are available with or without carry bags. Pump bag styles include shoulder bags and backpacks, and all bags include an insulated cooling compartment for milk storage during the work day. Most have battery options. Recommended brands include Ameda, Hygeia, and Medela (see the Resources section). Different mothers respond differently to the "feels" of various breast pump models (Kent, Ramsay, Doherty, Larsson, & Hartmann, 2003). That means there's not one pump make and model that works best for everyone

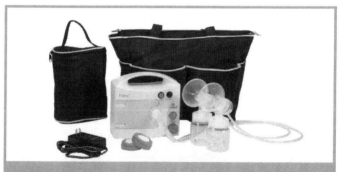

Figure 2. Professional-grade pumps are smaller and lighter than rental pumps. Most have battery options, carry bags, and compartments to store and cool milk. ©2014 Hygeia. Used with permission.

Some women get more milk per session with a manual pump than with an electric double pump, but because manual pumps require more muscle power, using them daily may not be practical long-term. If this is true for you, try the hands-on pumping technique described in the next chapter with an electric pump to increase your milk yield.

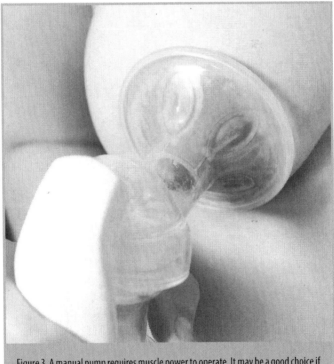

Figure 3. A manual pump requires muscle power to operate. It may be a good choice if you're not planning to pump every day.

You're Not Pumping Daily

If you work less than 20 hours per week, or you'll be breastfeeding your baby during your work day, you will not be relying as heavily on your breast pump to establish or maintain your milk production. This gives you many more options. Keep in mind that if you buy a single pump, pumping one breast at a time takes twice as long as double pumping. A manual pump, which is usually powered by squeezing the pump's handle, can get tiring if you use it often. Visit some of the many websites that compare breast-pump makes and models, and consider those with the features most important to you.

What about Used Breast Pumps?

Like many women, you may wonder if you can save money by getting a used breast pump. Here are the main points to ponder.

Rental and Purchase Pumps Differ

Some think that since mothers can safely share rental pumps, it is safe for them to share all other pumps. This is not true because these two types of pumps have different designs. Rental pumps are designed so your milk never touches the working parts of the pump that are shared with other mothers. The inner workings of most purchase pumps come in contact with milk particles during pumping, and there is no surefire way to avoid mixing milk.

Hygiene Issues

If you buy, borrow, or are given a used purchase pump, in most cases, it's impossible to prevent other mothers' milk particles from being blown into your milk during pumping. This is why some compare pumping with a used breast pump to sharing someone else's toothbrush.

With Medela double-electric purchase pumps, for example, the pump piece held against your breast is open to the pump's tubing, which is also open to the piece over the pump motor that generates the suction and release. This means that an invisible mist of milk particles can travel through the tubing to the inside of the pump. The piece inside the pump that the milk particles touch cannot be removed or sterilized, so it cannot be cleaned well enough between mothers to ensure safety—even with a new set of bottles and tubing. You may not see these milk particles, but they are the reason that mold sometimes grows in pump tubing. In contrast, Ameda's electric pumps are designed with a solid barrier between the milk and the pump tubing.

Wear and Tear

Another key consideration is whether a used pump will work well. Most rental pumps are bigger, heavier, and more durable than purchase pumps, which were designed to be used by one person only. Better double-electric purchase pumps have a one-year warranty on their motor, compared with a three-year warranty on most rental pumps.

If someone loans you her double-electric purchase pump, keep in mind that you will reduce its lifespan by however long you use it. Even if the original owner doesn't want the pump back, you have no way of knowing if it is still in good working order. If pumping is key to your milk production, starting with a new pump is a wise investment.

Pump Fit

If you'll be doing a lot of pumping, you'll want this time to be both productive and comfortable. Pump fit is key to both.

What Determines Pump Fit?

Pump fit is not about breast size; it's about nipple size. It refers to how well your nipples fit into the pump opening or "nipple tunnel" (Figure 4) that your nipple is pulled into during pumping.

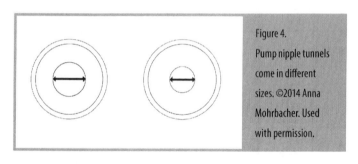

Figure 4. Pump nipple tunnels come in different sizes. ©2014 Anna Mohrbacher. Used with permission.

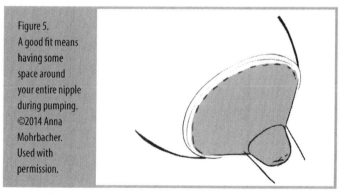

Figure 5. A good fit means having some space around your entire nipple during pumping. ©2014 Anna Mohrbacher. Used with permission.

You'll know you have a good pump fit if you see some (but not too much) space around your nipple as it moves freely in and out of the nipple tunnel (Figure 5).

If any part of your nipple rubs along the tunnel's sides, it is too small (Figure 6). It can also be too large. Ideally, you want no more than about a quarter inch (6 mm) of the dark circle around your nipple (areola) pulled into the tunnel during pumping.

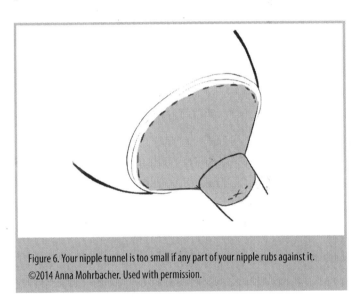

Figure 6. Your nipple tunnel is too small if any part of your nipple rubs against it. ©2014 Anna Mohrbacher. Used with permission.

Too much areola pulled into the tunnel can cause rubbing and soreness (Figure 7). You'll know you probably need a different size nipple tunnel if you feel discomfort during pumping, even when your pump's suction control is near its lowest setting.

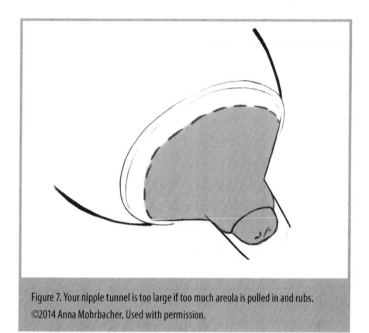

Figure 7. Your nipple tunnel is too large if too much areola is pulled in and rubs. ©2014 Anna Mohrbacher. Used with permission.

A good fit is important because it affects both your comfort and milk flow (Jones & Hilton, 2009). If the nipple tunnel squeezes your nipple during pumping, this slows your milk flow and you pump less milk. Either a too-large or too-small nipple tunnel can cause discomfort and stress, both of which also slow milk flow.

Available Sizes

Before getting a breast pump, find out how many size options the brand you're considering offers. If the only size option is the one that comes with the pump, you're taking a chance. Most companies that make quality breast pumps sell several nipple-tunnel sizes so that you can fit your pump to your anatomy.

The popular Medela and Ameda brands offer six or seven size options, and sell the part with the nipple tunnel separately, so if you need another size, you can buy just that piece. The Medela nipple-tunnel pieces are also compatible with the Hygeia brand pumps. However, some breast pump brands, such as Avent and Evenflo, sell only two sizes. Their pumps are packaged with an insert piece that you can either leave in or remove. With other breast pump brands, such as Playtex, the size that comes with the pump is the only size available.

Confused about where to start? Even before birth, you can use common objects to gauge which nipple-tunnel size you may want to try first. For example, hold a U.S. nickel up to your nipple. (If you live elsewhere, use any coin with a 22.5 mm diameter.) If your nipple width is larger than this, start with the next size up from standard. If your nipple is as wide as a U.S. quarter (25 mm) or larger, you may want to start with two sizes up from standard. On the other hand, if your nipple is smaller than a nickel (22.5 mm), start with the standard size that comes with the pump. However, if your nipple is quite a bit smaller than the nickel (perhaps the size of a pencil eraser), start with a smaller-than-standard size.

Because your nipples may vary in size, you may get better pumping results if you use a different nipple-tunnel size for each breast. The only way to know if the size you're using is the best fit for you is to experiment with several sizes. Some pumps come with multiple size options.

Pump Fit Changes Over Time

Once you find your best pump fit, that's not the end of the story. You need to recheck your fit now and then, because your nipples may expand with breast-feeding and pumping (Meier, Motykowski, & Zuleger, 2004). In other words, you may see space around your nipples now, but this space may eventually disappear. If your nipples begin to rub along your pump's nipple tunnel, don't be surprised. This just means it's time to switch to a larger size.

Pumping and Milk Expression

For many mothers, pumping is key to reaching their long-term breastfeeding goals. In spite of this higher purpose, pumping is not fun. In fact, it is the part of lactation many women hate most. One of the top four reasons mothers give for weaning earlier than planned is the time and work of pumping (Odom, Li, Scanlon, Perrine, & Grummer-Strawn, 2013). This chapter will give you tips to minimize the time you spend pumping and maximize your milk yields so that you have more time for those things that you do enjoy.

Realistic Pumping Expectations

Do you have specific ideas of how much milk you think you should be pumping? If so, you're not alone.

Unrealistic pumping expectations are the source of angst among many new mothers. Knowing what to expect can help you eliminate this item from your worry list.

What is the source of this worry? Many mothers compare their milk yield with the amount their friend or neighbor pumps, or they compare the milk they pump now with the milk they pumped for a previous baby. Before you judge your own results, you first need to know how much pumped milk is average. Many discover—to their surprise—that when they compare their own milk yields with the norm, they're doing just fine. Take a deep breath and read on.

Expect Less Milk during the First Month

If the first month of breastfeeding is going well and you're exclusively breastfeeding, your milk production dramatically increases from about 1 oz. (30 mL) on Day 1 to a peak of about 30 oz. (900 mL) per baby around Day 40. Draining your breasts well and often naturally boosts your milk during these early weeks. At first, while your milk production is ramping up, expect to pump less milk than you will later. If you pumped more milk for a previous child, you may be thinking back to a time when your milk production was already at its peak rather than during the early weeks while it was still building.

Practice Makes Perfect

What should you expect when you begin pumping? First know it takes time and practice to train your body to respond to your pump like it responds to your baby.

> "At first you will probably only pump small amounts of milk, which will gradually increase as time goes on."

At first you will probably only pump small amounts of milk, which will gradually increase as time goes on. Don't assume (as many do) that what you pump is a gauge of your milk production. That is rarely true, especially the first few times you pump. (Also, if you take a long break from pumping and then come back to it.) It takes time to become skilled at pumping. Even with good milk production and a good-quality pump, some mothers find pumping tricky at first.

How Many Minutes to Pump

Have you heard conflicting advice about how long to pump? This may not be a critical issue while you are practicing with your pump before going back to work or if you have plenty of milk stored. In some situations, though, how long you pump can be key. Examples are if you're trying to boost your supply or you're back at work and pumping to keep your milk supply stable. When deciding how many minutes to pump, remember that "drained breasts make milk faster" and "full breasts make milk slower."

Science recently shed new light on this issue. During pumping, researchers measured milk-flow rates among 34 women (Prime, Kent, Hepworth, Trengove, & Hartmann, 2012). They found great differences from mother to mother. Some pumped 60% of their available milk within the first minute and were done quickly, while others pumped as much as 20% of their milk 14 minutes into their session. The most helpful discovery was that although the women's experiences varied, each woman's milk-flow rates during pumping were consistent during different sessions. In other words, women who pumped their milk quickly did so at every pumping, as did women whose milk kept flowing for longer periods.

What does this tell us? Simply put, that it doesn't make sense to give all women a one-size-fits-all set of pumping guidelines based on averages. Rather, you can determine your own best pump time by watching what happens during two or three pump sessions. If you find you're still getting a fair amount of milk after 15 to 20 minutes, you should pump at least this long. But if you get nearly all of your milk within 5 minutes, you can stop after six or seven minutes. Let your milk flow be your guide. Keep in mind, though, that these study mothers used the breast pump alone to remove milk. Before settling on a routine, try the hands-on pumping technique described later.

Factors That Affect Milk Yield

After you've made sure you've got a good pump fit (see previous chapter), you've had some practice with your pump, and it's working well, the following factors may affect your milk yield:

- Your baby's age
- Whether or not you're exclusively breastfeeding
- Time elapsed since last breastfeeding or pumping
- Time of day
- Your emotional state
- Your breast storage capacity
- Your pump quality
- Your pump suction setting
- Whether or not you use your hands
- Number of milk releases

Here is what you need to know about each of these factors.

Your Baby's Age

How much milk a baby consumes per feeding varies by age and—until 1 month or so—by weight. Because newborns' stomachs are so small, during the first week most full-term babies take no more than 1 to 1.5 oz. (30 to 45 mL) at feedings. After about 4 to 5 weeks, babies reach their peak feeding volume of about 3 to 4 ounces (90 to 120 mL) and peak daily milk intake of about 25 to 30 ounces per day (750 to 900 mL).

Until your baby starts eating solid foods at around 6 months, her feeding volume and daily milk intake will not vary by much. Although babies get bigger and heavier between 1 and 6 months, their rate of growth slows down during that time, so the amount of milk they need per day stays about the same. This is not true for formula-fed babies, who consume much more as they grow. When your baby starts eating solid foods, her need for milk will gradually decrease as solids take your milk's place in her diet.

Exclusively Breastfeeding?

An exclusively breastfeeding baby receives only mother's milk (no other liquids or solids) primarily at the breast and is gaining weight well. A mother giving formula regularly will express less milk than an exclusively breastfeeding mother, because her milk production will be lower. If you're giving formula, and your baby is between 1 and 6 months old, you can calculate how much milk you should expect to pump at a session by determining what percentage of your baby's total daily intake is at the breast. To do this, subtract from 30 oz. (900 mL) the amount of formula your baby receives each day. For example, if you're giving 15 oz. (450 mL) of formula each day, this is half of 30 oz. (900 mL), so you should expect to pump about half of what an exclusively breastfeeding mother would pump.

Time Since Last Milk Removal

On average, if you're exclusively breastfeeding, had some practice with your pump, and it's working well for you, expect to pump:

- About half a feeding if you're pumping between regular feedings. After 1 month, this would be about 1.5 to 2 oz. (45 to 60 mL).

- A full feeding if you're pumping for a missed feeding. After one month, this would be about 3 to 4 oz. (90 to 120 mL).

Time of Day

Most women pump more milk in the morning than later in the day. That's because milk production varies during the day. To get the milk they need, many babies respond to this by simply breastfeeding more often when milk production is slower, usually in the afternoon and evening. A good time to pump milk to store is usually 30 to 60 minutes after the first morning nursing. Most mothers will pump more milk then than at other times. If you're an exception to this rule of thumb, pump whenever you get the best results.

Your Emotional State

If you feel upset, stressed, or angry when you sit down to pump, this releases adrenaline into your blood-stream, which can prevent your milk from flowing. If you're feeling bad and don't pump as much milk as usual, take a break and pump later, when you're feeling more relaxed.

Your Breast Storage Capacity

Your breast storage capacity is determined by the volume of milk available in your breasts during their fullest time of the day. Storage capacity is based on the amount of room in your milk-making glands, not breast size. It varies among mothers, and in the same mother from baby to baby. Your largest pumping milk yield can provide a clue to whether your storage capacity is large, medium, or small (Mohrbacher, 2011). Mothers with a larger storage capacity usually pump more milk in a session than mothers with a smaller storage capacity.

If your baby is at least 1 month old, you're exclusively breastfeeding, and pumping for a missed breastfeeding, a milk yield (from both breasts) of much more than about 4 oz. (120 mL) may indicate a large storage capacity. On the other hand, if you never pump more than 3 oz. (90 mL), even when it has been many hours since your last milk removal, your storage capacity may be smaller.

What matters to your baby is not how much milk she gets at each feeding, but how much milk she receives over a 24-hour day. Breast storage capacity explains many of the differences in breastfeeding patterns and pump yields that are common among mothers.

Your Pump Quality

For most mothers, automatic double pumps that generate between 40 and 60 suction-and-release cycles per minute are most effective at expressing milk. This includes the rental pumps and professional-grade pumps described in the previous chapter.

Your Pump Suction Setting

Does common sense tell you that stronger suction will pump more milk? Not so. If your suction is set too high, discomfort (which can cause you to tense up) can actually prevent your milk from flowing. The best setting is the highest that's truly comfortable and no higher (Kent et al., 2008). This setting will vary among mothers, at different times, and could be anywhere on your pump's controls.

To find your highest comfortable setting, turn up your pump's suction until it feels slightly uncomfortable and then turn it down a little. Some mothers pump the most milk near the pump's minimum suction setting. A higher suction setting may be comfortable after your milk starts flowing, so try re-adjusting it upward, then see.

Whether or Not You Use Your Hands

"...a study found that mothers got 48% more milk when they used their hands while pumping"

Until recent years, we thought the breast pump should do all of the milk-removal work. Then a study found that mothers got 48% more milk when they used their hands while pumping (Morton et al., 2009). How does this technique, known as "hands-on pumping," work? Follow these steps:

1. First, massage both breasts.

2. Double-pump (pump both breasts at the same time), compressing your breasts often while pumping. Continue until milk flow slows to a trickle.

3. Stop pumping and massage your brea
concentrating on areas that feel full.

4. Finish by either hand-expressing your milk into the pump's nipple tunnel or by single-pumping, whichever yields the most milk. Either way, during this step, do intensive breast compression on each breast, moving back and forth from breast to breast several times until you've drained both breasts as fully as possible.

For the mothers in the study, this pumping routine took on average about 25 minutes total. For an online demonstration video, see "How to Use Your Hands When You Pump" at this website: _newborns.stanford.edu/ Breastfeeding/MaxProduction.html_. Another plus of using the hands-on pumping technique is that it drains your breasts more fully, maintaining milk supply better and doubling milk-fat content (Morton et al., 2012).

Number of Milk Releases

As mentioned, stronger suction does not necessarily yield more milk. Why not? Because the key to effective milk expression is a muscle action known as let-down, milk ejection, or milk release. The number of milk releases you have during pumping can have a major effect on your milk yield.

Milk Release Is Key

What is a milk release? It is triggered by the hormone oxytocin, which causes the muscles inside the breast to squeeze your milk-making glands and push the milk out. Without it, most milk stays in your breast.

Some mothers feel milk release as a tingling sensation or see it as leaking milk, while others feel and see nothing. By watching your milk flow during pumping, you will see your milk releases as an obviously faster milk flow. During breastfeeding, you can hear milk releases when your baby begins gulping.

The fewer milk releases triggered during pumping, the less milk you'll pump. With no milk release, you'll express only the small amount of milk pooled around your nipples, which is at most about half an ounce (15 mL) per breast. This is one reason pumping isn't an accurate gauge of your milk production.

Without even realizing it, most mothers average about five milk releases at each breastfeeding (Prime et al., 2012). Some feel the first milk release, but very few feel those that come later (Geddes, 2009). Some mothers feel none. Even if you don't feel a milk release, your baby's swallowing and weight gain tell you they're happening.

While your baby is at the breast, milk release is triggered by her suckling, the feel of her soft skin against yours, her warmth, and your loving thoughts. Even when your baby is not breastfeeding, a milk release can happen when your breasts are touched, you hear your baby (or another baby!) cry, even when you think about your baby. Feelings of tension, anger, or frustration can block it.

When you pump, your baby's softness and warmth are missing. Suction from a piece of plastic feels very different from your baby's warm mouth and tongue. As you train your body to respond to the feel of the pump, you may need extra help to trigger milk releases. You may also need extra help when you switch from one pump to another, because the new pump has a different feel than the old pump. Mothers who have a regular pumping routine often say that following this routine is part of conditioning their body to release milk. The next section provides some tips for triggering more milk releases during pumping, which may increase your milk yields.

If you need help releasing your milk to the pump, try the following suggestions.

Use Your Senses

You can experiment with your senses to help condition your body to release your milk to the feel of the pump.

- **Feelings:** Get comfortable. Pump in a private place where you can relax. Close your eyes and imagine your baby at your breast. Breathe deeply and imagine a tranquil setting.

- **Sight:** Look at your baby or your baby's photo. Play a video of her.

- **Hearing:** Play an audio or video recording of your baby cooing or crying. Call to check on your baby, or call someone you love to relax and distract you.

- **Smell:** Smell your baby's blanket or clothing while you pump.

- **Touch:** Gently massage your breasts or apply warm compresses.

- **Taste:** Sip a favorite warm drink to relax you.

As needed, use whichever of your senses work best. Within a short time, you can condition your body to respond to the feel of your pump. You can also use these strategies whenever you're feeling stressed.

Vary Your Pump Speed

Most babies suckle faster at first to trigger milk release and then use slower jaw movements while the milk is flowing to drain the breast faster. If your pump has a speed or cycle control, try this approach to mimic your baby's rhythm.

- Start pumping on the "fast" setting.

- When milk starts flowing, go to a "slow" setting.

- Return to "fast" after milk flow slows or stops.

- Repeat until you see at least three to five milk releases.

If you have a two-phase pump with a let-down button, be aware that these pumps are programmed to automatically switch from a fast to slow speed after two minutes. That's how long it takes on average for a milk release to occur. If your body takes more or less time to let-down your milk, you can customize the pump to work better for you. For example, if your milk release occurs before two minutes, press this button to switch to a slower speed as soon as it happens. Then return to a faster speed when your milk release ends and milk flow slows. You can use the let-down button several times during the pumping to speed up the milk-removal process. Your baby would do this automatically, but you can mimic this pattern by adjusting your pump according to your milk flow.

Double-Pumping: One Handed or Hands Free

Women often wonder how they're supposed to adjust their pump controls while double pumping. Are three hands required? Thankfully, no.

There are also many hands-free double-pumping options. Some pumps are marketed as hands-free pumps. The most costly models include bands and fasteners that make this process more difficult than it needs to be. Almost any double-electric pump can easily be converted to a hands-free pump with the right accessories. You don't need to overspend on your breast pump to pump hands free. For the most up-to-date listing of retail pumping bras and bustiers (bands that fit over your bra with button holes to hold your pump parts in place), do an internet search for "hands-free pumping."

There are also creative, lower-cost options. Some women buy inexpensive stretchy sports bras and cut holes in them to insert the pump pieces. Here are two internet tutorials on homemade options that use elastic hair bands and rubber bands:

- *http://kellymom.com/bf/pumpingmoms/pumping/hands-free-pumping/*

- *http://www.workandpump.com/handsfree.htm (be sure to click on the photos)*

If you'll be spending lots of time pumping, it makes sense to make it as easy as possible.

Forgot Your Pump or Parts?

Sooner or later, nearly every pumping mother leaves something at home that's key to pumping. Here are some ways to plan ahead or handle it on the spot.

Bottles

- Keep a package of milk storage bags with your things at work and attach them to your pump parts with rubber bands.

- Go to the closest grocery or drugstore and buy standard-sized bottles of any size. Wash with hot, soapy water and rinse well before using, or buy some steam sterilizer bags and sanitize it in your workplace microwave.

Pump Left Behind or Useless Due to Missing Parts

- Keep a good manual pump with your things at work in case of emergency.

- Go to the closest baby store and buy a good manual pump. Either wash it in hot, soapy water and rinse well before using, or buy some steam sterilizer bags and sanitize it in your workplace microwave.

- Hand express your milk (see Appendix B) into any clean, wide-mouthed container.

- If missing parts, see if they're available to buy at the closest baby store or hospital gift shop.

Freezer Packs

- Keep your milk in the work refrigerator.

- Use ice sealed in Ziploc bags until you get home.

- In the pain relief section of the drugstore, look for cold packs used for sports injuries that chill when a seal is broken.

- See Table 1 for safe storage times at different room-temperature ranges.

What If Pumping Hurts?

"No pain, no gain" does not apply to pumping. Just like during breastfeeding, pain while pumping is a sign that some adjustment is needed. If pumping is painful, consider these possibilities.

If you'll be spending lots of time pumping, it makes sense to make it as easy as possible.

Pump Suction Set Too High

As mentioned before, the highest suction setting does not always pump the most milk. Set your pump at the highest suction level that feels comfortable during and after pumping...and no higher. For some, this might be the minimum pump setting. Don't push the envelope. If you're gritting your teeth, it's too high!

Pump Doesn't Fit

Many mothers pump comfortably with the standard diameter nipple tunnel that comes with their pump. But if pumping hurts even on low suction, you most likely need another size. To check your pump fit, see Chapter 2.

Breast or Nipple Health Issues

If your pain is not due to too-high suction, or too-small or too-large nipple tunnels, ask yourself these questions. Do you have (or have you had) nipple trauma? If you had nipple trauma in the past, could you have developed a bacterial infection of the nipple? Do you have an overgrowth of yeast (also known as thrush or candida)? Could you have mastitis? Does your nipple turn white, red, or blue after pumping? If it does, see your lactation consultant or other health care provider to rule out the circulatory problem Raynaud's Phenomenon and other causes related to breast and nipple health. Pumping pain may be a sign of a condition that needs to be treated.

The Feel of Hard Plastic

Some women find the feel of hard plastic on their breasts uncomfortable. If none of the above tips help, try using a soft pumping insert or a different style nipple-tunnel piece (one that some mothers find more comfortable is the Pumpin' Pal at *www.pumpinpal.com*).

Both Avent and Playtex pumps come with a soft silicone insert. Or you can buy soft inserts separately and try them with your pump. Options include the Avent Isis Petal Massager and the Ameda Flexishield Areola Stimulator. The Ameda Flexishield Areola Stimulator narrows your nipple tunnel to its smallest size of 21 mm, so this won't be a good choice unless you have very small nipples.

Less-Than-Average Milk Yield

Breast pumps work well for the vast majority of women, but there are exceptions. If your baby is gaining well and you are breastfeeding exclusively, you know your milk production is not the problem. But if you've tried hands-on pumping and all of the other suggestions for improving milk yield in this chapter and you're still unable to pump even average milk volumes, it's time to try a different approach.

One option is to switch from a purchase pump to a rental pump. Some mothers get much better results with the types of pumps used in hospitals. To find one, visit the websites of Ameda, Hygeia, and Medela, which feature locators for local pump rental stations.

Another alternative is a time-tested approach used all over the world: hand expression. For some women, the skin-to-skin contact of hand expression greatly improves milk yield. In some cases, the pumping problem is due to unusual breast anatomy. The pump parts don't come in contact with the areas needed to effectively pump milk. Hand expression is a learned skill, but with practice, many women learn to do it quickly and efficiently.

4

Hand Expressing Milk

Hand expression can be a useful way to relieve breast fullness, boost milk production, and provide milk for your baby. Here's how to do it.

Getting ready

First, wash your hands well. Find a clean collection container with a wide mouth, like a cup. If possible, express in a private, comfortable place where you can relax. Feeling relaxed enhances milk flow.

Find your sweet spot

Whichever hand-expression technique you use, the key is finding your "sweet spot," the area on your breast where milk flows fastest when it is compressed. Try different finger positions until you find it. If the dark area around your nipple (areola) is large, your sweet spot may be inside it. If it is small, your sweet spot may be outside it.

Do what works best and expresses the most milk

This method combines the World Health Organization technique with others:

1. Before expressing, gently massage your breasts with your hands and fingertips or a soft baby brush or warm towel.

2. Sit up and lean slightly forward, so gravity helps milk flow.

3. To find your sweet spot, start with your thumb on top of the breast and fingers below, both about 1.5 inches (4 cm) from the base of the nipple. Some mothers find it helpful to curl their hand and use just the tips of their fingers and thumb. Apply steady pressure several times into the breast toward the chest wall. If no milk comes, shift finger and thumb either closer to or farther from the nipple and compress again a few times. Repeat, moving finger and thumb until you feel slightly firmer

breast tissue and gentle pressure yields milk. After finding your sweet spot, skip the "finding" phase and start with your fingers on this area.

4. Apply steady pressure on areas of milk in the breast by pressing fingers toward the chest wall, not toward the nipple.

5. While applying inward pressure on the breast, compress thumb and finger pads together (pushing in, not pulling out toward the nipple). Find a good rhythm of press—compress—relax, like a baby's suckling rhythm.

6. Switch breasts every few minutes (5 or 6 times in total at each expression) while rotating finger position around the breast. After expressing, all areas of the breast should feel soft. This process usually takes about 20 to 30 minutes.

If needed, adjust

Hand expression should feel comfortable. If not, you may be compressing too hard, sliding your fingers along the skin, or squeezing the nipple. If you feel discomfort, review the instructions, and adjust your technique. It is important to find the method that works best for you. You can find several demonstration videos online by doing a search for "hand expression of breast milk."

5

Milk Storage and Handling

Most mothers—whether employed or not—have questions about how to store and handle their milk. This chapter covers most of the basics, as well as some not-so-basic situations. It includes storage and handling options when traveling without your baby, which is part of some jobs. It also explains why some women's frozen milk develops a soapy taste (or worse), what you need to know about this, and how to prevent it.

What Your Milk Looks Like

You may be concerned the first time you notice your expressed milk looks very different from the cow's milk in the dairy case. Knowing why it looks different, and what to expect, may help set your mind at ease.

Layers

Over time, your pumped milk naturally separates into layers of milk and cream. Commercially sold cow's milk is homogenized, a process that prevents this separation from happening. Because your milk is not homogenized, expect that as it sits, layers will form. If these layers are obvious, before feeding your milk to your baby, gently swirl your milk, so that the cream mixes with the milk. This prevents the cream (which contains most of the milk fat) from being left on the sides of your container.

Colors

Expect color variations in your milk as time passes and with changes in your diet. During the first two to three weeks after birth, your milk is likely to be yellower than it will be later. In the last half of pregnancy and the first few days after birth, your breasts make colostrum (the concentrated first milk), which is often yellow or gold, but sometimes looks clear. As your milk increases in volume on the third or fourth day, it becomes transitional milk, a mixture of mature milk and colostrum. Finally, after the first two or three weeks, your milk is considered mature. At this stage, mature milk may appear bluish, yellowish, or even brownish in color.

Many women wonder if it is all right to feed their baby with milk pumped at a different stage of lactation.

This concern is easy to answer. As long as you follow the milk-storage guidelines, your milk will always be a good choice, even if you give early milk to an older child.

Some foods, food dyes, and medications can change the color of your milk (Lawrence & Lawrence, 2011). If you eat or drink something containing orange food coloring, for example, such as orange soda or gelatin, your milk may look a little pink or pink-orange. If you eat a large amount of kelp, or guzzle many green drinks, your milk may have a greenish tinge. If you've taken the antibiotic minocycline, your milk may even look black. Frozen milk may take on a yellowish hue, but it is not spoiled unless it smells or tastes sour.

It is not uncommon for your milk to have a reddish tinge during the early weeks. One study found that 15% of new mothers had red blood cells in their milk (Kline & Lash, 1964). Sometimes called "rusty-pipe syndrome," blood in the milk may be due to the extra blood flow to the breast, and the fast increase in milk production after birth. It is not a cause for concern and should disappear within a few weeks (Mohrbacher, 2010). Blood and milk have many of the same ingredients, and it is not only safe for your baby to drink this milk, it is head-and-shoulders better for your baby than nonhuman milks.

Milk-Storage Strategies and Guidelines

There's a lot to know about storing and handling your milk. This section covers best practices and explains why some milk-storage strategies are better than others.

Storage Strategies

When you're ready to start expressing your milk, review these recommended storage strategies.

How Much Milk Per Container?

Ideally, you want to store milk in the smallest volume you think your baby might take. The closer you can get to your baby's actual intake, the less waste there will be. You can always add more milk to a container, but because your milk mixes with your baby's saliva during feedings, most recommend that any milk left after feedings be discarded. (For more, see the section "Milk Left After Feeding" later in this chapter.)

Fresh, Refrigerated, or Frozen

If your baby gets most of his milk directly from the breast, you don't need to worry about whether the relatively small amount of pumped milk he gets is fresh, refrigerated, or previously frozen. However, if a substantial percentage of your baby's daily milk intake is expressed milk, consider more carefully your milk-storage choices.

Freezing kills the live cells in the milk, which help keep your baby healthy. So if a significant amount of your baby's daily milk intake is expressed milk, rather than freezing all of your pumped milk and using the oldest milk first, plan to feed your baby as much fresh or refrigerated milk as possible. This might mean keeping your freezer stash for emergencies and leaving what you pump each day at work for the next day's feedings.

Choosing Storage Containers

Does it matter what kind of milk-storage containers you use? In general, any food-grade container with a tight-fitting, solid lid (rather than one with a feeding nipple attached) can be used to store expressed milk.

There have been few studies done on container materials, and many of their conclusions are conflicting. This means that aside from stainless steel, which is not recommended because fewer live cells survive, there is no definitive best choice (Manohar, Williamson, & Koppikar, 1997; Williamson & Murti, 1996). One study found that more of one milk component (leukocytes) adhered to glass rather than plastic, which led to the recommendation that fresh milk be stored in plastic (Paxson & Cress, 1979). A second study found that different types of leukocytes react differently to glass (Pittard & Bill, 1981). A third study found that over time many of the leukocytes were released from the glass, and after 24 hours milk stored in glass had more leukocytes than the milk stored in plastic (Goldblum, Garza, Johnson, Harrist, & Nichols, 1981). Some recommend glass as a good first choice for freezing milk because it is the least porous, thus providing the best protection.

Avoid storing milk in polycarbonate plastic containers, which contain the chemical bisphenol-A (BPA). There are concerns that under certain conditions, this chemical could leach into the milk, and it is associated with possible health risks. As of this writing, however, polypropylene plastic is considered safe for milk storage.

Milk freezer bags have some practical advantages over hard-sized containers. They take up less storage space and can be attached directly to breast pump attachments in place of bottles. Because they are not reused, there is less to wash, but that makes them less eco-friendly. A 2013 study found that it's better to use glass containers rather than polyethylene milk bags for refrigerated milk because the bactericidal activity of the milk (which prevents spoiling) is better maintained in glass (Takci, Gulmez, Yigit, Dogan, & Hascelik, 2013).

Some types of milk bags are not recommended. Bags intended to be used as "bottle liners" are made mainly for feeding rather than milk storage, and tend to be thinner and more prone to splitting. If you use this type of bag, to safeguard your milk, insert your bag of milk inside another bag (double-bag it) before sealing and storing. Plastic sandwich bags are not recommended because they are thin and tear easily.

Because there is no one overwhelmingly best choice when it comes to milk-storage containers, feel free to use whichever option is most practical for you.

Why Milk Storage Guidelines Differ

It can be really unsettling to read different milk-storage guidelines in different places. Why do guidelines differ, and why can't the experts agree amongst themselves? There's actually a simple explanation.

Take a look at the milk-storage times in Table 1. Some are listed as "Okay" while others are labeled "Ideal." Within the "Okay" time ranges, pumped milk should not go bad. Over time, however, even though the milk is not spoiled, more vitamins, antioxidants, and immunological factors are lost. The shorter storage times labeled "Ideal" are the guidelines some organizations recommend because fewer of these milk components are lost.

The takeaway message is that while it is always better to use your milk sooner rather than later, your milk should not spoil if you store it within the "Okay" time frames. Stored milk that you find in the back of the fridge that has been there for up to eight days will still be far better for your baby than formula.

Some milk-storage guidelines also vary because they define "room temperature" differently. If you live in a subtropical climate, for example, the higher room-temperature range in Table 1 may be closer to your experience. But if you live in a more temperate clime, the lower range may be closer to yours.

You may have noticed that refrigerator storage times for fresh and refrigerated milk are longer than those for previously frozen milk. They differ because freezing kills the live cells in the milk, making the milk more susceptible to spoilage.

When in doubt about the freshness of your milk, smell or taste it. Spoiled milk will smell spoiled.

Storage Guidelines for Full-term Healthy Babies at Home

The guidelines in Table 1 are specifically for full-term, healthy babies at home. If your baby is hospitalized, the time frames your hospital gives you are likely to be shorter. Preterm and ill babies are at greater risk for serious health problems, so your hospital may recommend you use stricter hygiene, such as storing your milk in sterile containers, or boiling your pump parts regularly.

These guidelines offer more options than many mothers realize. For example, you can refrigerate

Table 1. IMilk Storage Guidelines

Temperature	Deep Freezer (0°F/-18°C)	Refrigerator Freezer (variable) (0°F/-18°C)	Refrigerator (39°F/4°C)	Insulated Cooler with Ice Packs (59°F/15°C)	Room Temperature (66°F-72°F/19°C-22°C)	(73°F-77°F/23°C-25°C)
Fresh	Ideal: 6 mos. Okay: 12 mos.	3-4 mos.	Ideal: 72 hrs. Okay: 8 days	24 hrs.	6-10 hrs.	4 hrs.
Frozen Thawed in Fridge	Do not refreeze	Do not refreeze	24 hrs.	Do not Store	4 hrs.	4hrs.
Thawed, Warmed, Not Fed	Do not refreeze	Do not refreeze	4 hrs.	Do not Store	Until feeding ends	Until feeding ends
Warmed, Fed	Discard	Discard	Discard	Discard	Until Feeding ends	Until feeding ends

room-temperature milk at any point before its time is up. Depending on your room temperature, this would be before four hours (66°F to 72°F or 19°C to 22°C) or before six to 10 hours (73°F to 77°F or 23°C to 25°C). You can freeze refrigerated milk any time before eight days.

Power Failures and Freezer Stashes

Power failures are not uncommon. If you have a large freezer stash of expressed milk, you may worry about what will happen if a major storm or a power-grid failure cuts off power to your freezer for an extended time. If you find yourself in that situation, and you think the power failure will be short term, keep the freezer door closed to keep temperatures low for as long as possible. If your milk stays frozen, there's no issue. If it's possible to move your milk to a working freezer, consider doing so.

As you can see from Table 1, current guidelines recommend not refreezing thawed milk. Ideally, if your milk thaws, you will use that milk within 24 hours. But what if that's not possible? Do you really need to discard your milk?

Before tossing your milk, you should know the results of a study that examined the effects of refreezing donor milk expressed with normal hygiene (Rechtman, Lee, & Berg, 2006). The frozen milk was thawed at refrigerator temperature (39°F /4°C) overnight, separated into different sample batches, and refrozen to -80°C (-110°F). These sample batches were later thawed to room temperature (73°F/23°C), and each batch exposed to one of the following conditions: 46°F (8°C) for 8 or 24 hours, 73°F (23°C) for 4 or 8 hours, multiple freeze-thaw cycles of varying lengths, and the control batch kept at a steady -4°F (-20°C).

Bottom line, none of the batches developed unacceptable bacterial counts, and vitamin content remained at adequate levels. After this research was published, official milk-storage guidelines were not changed. In the case of a power failure, as you weigh your options, this information may provide some helpful perspective.

Safely Handling Your Milk

When you go to the trouble of pumping your milk, you want to make sure it stays as safe and nutritious as possible. The recommendations in this section will help you meet this goal.

Combining Batches

One of the most commonly asked questions about milk handling is whether you can combine the milk from one pumping session with another. Some mothers even ask whether it's okay when double-pumping (pumping both breasts at once) to combine the milk from the two containers afterwards. The answer to both questions is "yes."

If you add milk from your current pumping session to the milk from previous sessions, just make sure to date the milk according to the oldest batch. For example, if you add milk expressed on May 11 to refrigerated milk from May 10, the combined batch should be dated May 10.

Fresh milk can be added directly to refrigerated milk without cooling it first. Fresh milk can also be added to frozen milk, as long as there is less fresh milk than frozen milk, and it is first cooled for about an hour so that it does not thaw the top layer.

Thawing Frozen Milk

The best way to thaw frozen milk is by warming it gently and gradually, keeping heat low. Then swirl the milk to mix layers rather than shaking it. Freezing and heating your milk destroys some of its immune properties that kill bacteria, making it more vulnerable to contamination.

Milk can be thawed in the refrigerator overnight. Once thawed, it will be good in the fridge for up to 24 hours. You can also thaw or warm milk in other ways.

- Hold the container under cool running water for a few minutes.

- Hold the container in water previously heated on the stove. If the water cools and the milk is not yet thawed, remove the container of milk and reheat the water. Do not heat the milk on the stove burner directly.

If you use water to thaw or warm milk, tilt or hold the container, so the water cannot seep under the lid. Plan to feed thawed milk right away or refrigerate it (Jones & Tully, 2011).

Warming Milk for Feeding

When your baby is a newborn, it is best to warm your expressed milk to between room and body temperature before feeding. Older babies may drink chilled milk directly from the refrigerator. But for a small baby, cold milk can lower body temperature. Use either warm, running water or water warmed on the stove to gently heat milk for feeding.

Microwaves Are a No-No

A microwave should not be used to thaw or warm your milk. Why? Because it changes your milk's components and destroys much of its anti-infective factors (Quan et al., 1992). Microwaves also heat liquids unevenly, so even if afterwards the milk is swirled (or even shaken), hot spots remain that can burn your baby's throat.

Milk Left After Feeding

Most guidelines recommend discarding any milk left after a feeding because the milk mixes with the baby's saliva. La Leche League International is the exception: its milk-storage handout says that leftover milk can be used, but only at the next feeding (LLLI, 2008).

No published studies have scientifically examined the safety of feeding leftover milk, but a college student researched this scenario for her unpublished senior thesis (Brusseau, 1998). In her study, she divided fresh milk donated from six women into two bottles, one of which was warmed and partially fed to their babies. The leftover milk and the milk in the bottle not fed (the control milk) were cultured right after feeding and again 12, 24, 36, and 48 hours later. The only milk with higher bacterial counts was one batch of the warmed and fed milk from a mother who had not followed instructions, and had donated previously frozen instead of fresh milk. All other batches of milk showed no change in total bacterial counts within 48 hours after feeding.

This is an issue that affects many families, and there is little science behind the current recommendations. Hopefully, this information will help you make up your own mind about how best to handle your leftover milk.

Your Milk Is Not a Biohazard

It bears mentioning that one type of push-back related to milk storage and handling that employed mothers in the past have dealt with (and that we've hopefully moved beyond) is the fear that because mother's milk is a body fluid, it should be treated as a biohazard. American agencies and organizations, such as the Occupational Safety and Health Administration, the American Academy of Pediatrics, and the Centers for Disease Control and Prevention have issued statements confirming that human milk is not a biohazardous substance, and no gloves or other special precautions are needed when handling it: *http://www.cdc.gov/breastfeeding/disease/hiv.htm.* At workplaces and childcare facilities, your milk can be stored with other foods in a common refrigerator with no special precautions needed.

Options When Traveling Without Your Baby

Some mothers have the option of bringing their babies along when they travel, and some don't. If you'll be traveling without your baby, either for work or for personal reasons, see the previous chapter for recommendations on how often to pump. Regarding what to do with your pumped milk while you're traveling, you have several choices.

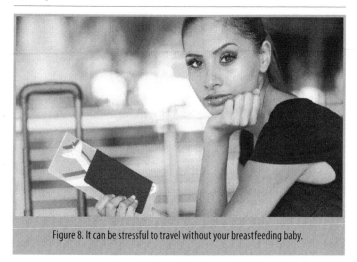

Figure 8. It can be stressful to travel without your breastfeeding baby.

Pump and Dump

Pouring your expressed milk down the drain is painful for sure, even if you have a lot of extra milk at home. If you have access to a refrigerator at your destination, keep in mind that your milk will be good there for up to eight days.

> While traveling, if you won't have easy access to a freezer to chill your pump case's cooling elements at night, bring many Ziploc bags with you to fill with ice and keep your milk cool. When it's time to travel home, you can also seal your milk containers in these bags to prevent leaking in transit.

Hand Carry Milk Home

When traveling home, you can hand-carry at least some of your milk home in your pump's cooling compartment and/or another cooler carrier. Your milk is good for at least 10 hours this way, and when you get it home you can then either refrigerate or freeze it.

In the U.S., see current Transportation Security Administration regulations on traveling by air with mother's milk at: _http://www.tsa.gov/traveling-formula-breast-milk-and-juice_. Here is a January 2014 excerpt from their website:

> When carrying breast milk through security check-points, it is treated in the same manner as liquid medication. Parents flying with, and without, their child(ren) are permitted to bring breast milk in quantities greater than three ounces as long as it is presented for inspection at the security checkpoint.

When traveling by air, it may be helpful to bring a printed copy of the current guidelines to share with airport security if needed.

Ship Milk Home

A third option is to freeze your milk while you're away and ship it home. Obviously, access to a freezer at your destination is a must. If you are traveling for work, some companies will cover these shipping costs, which are not small. For recommendations on how to safely ship frozen milk from point A to point B, see: _http://newborns.stanford.edu/Breastfeeding/ShipNStore.html_.

Stored Milk That Smells Soapy or Rancid

Before amassing a huge reserve of frozen milk, it's a good idea to freeze several batches of your milk, thaw them after about a week, and then smell them.

Soapy-Smelling Milk

Some mothers make milk that has higher-than-average levels of the enzyme lipase, which over time, breaks down fat in expressed milk. This fat breakdown can cause cooled or frozen milk to develop a soapy smell and taste. Depending on the level of lipase in your milk, this change in smell and/or taste may occur sooner or later. Freezing slows but does not stop lipase from digesting the milk fat.

Safe for babies. This soapy-tasting milk is safe for babies, and many babies will drink this milk without a problem (Lawrence & Lawrence, 2011). Megan B. from Illinois USA returned to work full-time as a sales operations manager for a travel gear company when her son was 3 months old. She didn't realize until later in lactation that her milk was high in lipase, because it didn't affect her or her baby.

> "I didn't really know [my milk] was high lipase un-
> til just recently. My son drank the milk fine. It just
> had a soapy smell."

When it's a problem. This becomes a serious issue,

though, if the baby will not accept the soapy-tasting milk. Marissa S. from Pennsylvania, USA describes an experience no mother wants to go through.

> "I remember crying when I had to throw away my freezer stash three days before returning to work. I was definitely not prepared for it!"

What you can do about it. The purpose of freezing a few batches for a week or more, and testing them for this soapy smell or taste is to avoid the need to discard a huge reserve of frozen milk. (Read on for other alternatives.) If your milk develops this soapy smell or taste and your baby accepts it, no problem. But if your baby doesn't accept it, what's next? Once your milk-fat is broken down, this process cannot be reversed.

If you find out in advance that high lipase levels may be an issue for you (mothers report their milk's lipase levels can vary from baby to baby), one approach is to scald your milk before chilling or freezing it to deactivate the lipase and prevent this fat breakdown from occurring. Heating your milk is not routinely recommended, because it kills live cells in the milk. But if your baby will not accept your pumped milk otherwise, this makes it possible for your milk to be used (Jones & Tully, 2011). How should you scald your milk?

- Heat your milk in a pan on the stove until small bubbles form around the edges, but it is not yet at a full boil.

- Cool it quickly.

Jenn G., a full-time special-education teacher from South Carolina, USA, found herself in this situation.

Soon after giving birth, I started pumping, as I was going back to work when my daughter was 18 weeks old. After 14 weeks of pumping and feeding on demand, I had nearly 300 oz. (9000 mL) of breast milk stored. It was around this time that I offered my daughter a frozen bottle of milk. She refused it. I offered a second bottle, and she refused that. I smelled the milk, and it had a very soapy smell to it. I, of course, looked that up right away on Google and read about lipase. I thawed three more bags of milk, they all had that smell, and she refused them. So here I was about four weeks before returning to work with no useable milk, even though I had nearly 275 oz. (8250 mL) in my freezer.

I quickly learned that I would need to scald my milk. I took 5 oz. (150 mL) of freshly pumped milk and put in into five one-ounce bottles. I checked each bottle every five hours to see when my milk started to taste and smell bad. I found out that it was around hour 26. So I knew I could get through my entire school day without having to scald it at school. As soon as I got home each day, I began what my family affectionately called my science-fair experiment. I would scald all my milk. Then I would quickly put it all in glass bottles and cool it.

Not every mother with high milk lipase levels scalds her milk. Serena C. from Montana, USA structured her day so that she could exclusively breastfeed without using frozen milk at all.

> We found ways around, it including breastfeeding on my lunch break, and then sending home the earlier pumped milk for later, as well as some reverse cycling. I ended up donating my whole freezer stash to a milk bank.

If this extra work concerns you, it may help to know how others have either fit scalding their milk into their busy lives or found ways to reduce the need for it.

When Michelle R. from Wisconsin, USA, a full-time teacher, discovered that her milk was high in lipase and her freezer reserve had gone "bad," she did some online research and some experiments.

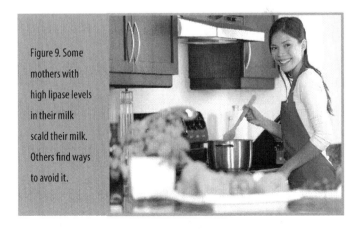

Figure 9. Some mothers with high lipase levels in their milk scald their milk. Others find ways to avoid it.

She found that in her case, it took three days for the change in smell and taste to occur, and she felt overwhelmed at first. "Didn't I already have enough to deal with: working full-time, pumping, and then being a mama the rest of the time?" But she soldiered on and discovered that she only needed to scald her milk once a week.

> I developed a system where I used that day's fresh milk for the next day's daycare supply. On Friday, I would collect the milk and scald it in a pot, place the pot on ice just until it cooled, and finally pour it into storage bags. Come Sunday night, I would place those bags in the fridge to prepare for Monday at daycare. I felt very fortunate that I only had to do this on Fridays.

The previous mothers who shared their stories either donated their soapy-smelling milk to a milk bank or discarded it. But if you discover your milk has developed a soapy smell, before getting rid of it, know that there may be ways to use it even after the fat breakdown has occurred.

Some mothers find that their baby will take soapy-smelling milk if it is mixed with fresh or refrigerated milk. If you decide to use some of this milk, what ratio of soapy milk to fresh milk will make it acceptable to your baby? This varies by lipase level and by the baby. To find your best ratio of soapy-smelling milk to refrigerated milk, start with a half-and-half mixture. If the baby accepts that, you may want to try two-thirds to one third. Keep experimenting until you find the most soapy-tasting milk per container your baby will accept. That will allow you to use your freezer stash rather than pouring it down the drain.

Some sensitive babies even refuse milk that has been scalded. Marissa S., a full-time behavior specialist from Pennsylvania, USA, was extremely stressed when she found out that three days before going back to work that her baby refused her stored milk. By adding it to fresh milk, she found a way around it.

One thing I found out through trial and error was that if my pumped milk was fed within 24 hours, the fats did not break down too much and my daughter would still drink it. When I knew I would need to refrigerate or freeze my milk for more than a day, that night I would scald it before bed, and make sure to label everything clearly so that I could use the oldest first. I found my picky daughter really didn't like the scalded milk much, so I would freeze them in one-ounce stick forms to add an ounce or two to fresh bottles as needed, which she tolerated much better. I was the only person who did the scalding, as it is such a delicate process, and I didn't want to put the stress on my husband. I knew I would've been upset if the milk was over-processed.

These mothers did the scalding themselves. But in some families, the mother's partner could take on this task.

Sour or Rancid-Smelling Milk

If you use the milk-storage guidelines in Table 1 to store your milk and it becomes sour or rancid-smelling within its time frames, this change is probably unrelated to spoilage or milk-lipase levels. According to some food-storage experts, the most likely cause is chemical oxidation (Jones & Tully, 2011). One way to know if chemical oxidation is the cause is to scald some batches of your freshly pumped milk before freezing or cooling it (see previous section). In this case, heating will speed this breakdown, making the smell worse instead of better.

If sour or rancid-smelling milk is an issue for you, you may be able to prevent this change by avoiding free copper or iron ions in your water and polyunsaturated fats in your diet. Here are some specific changes that may help.

- Avoid drinking your local tap water; switch to bottled water for a while.

- Stop taking any fish-oil or flaxseed supplements.

- Avoid any foods, like anchovies, that contain rancid fats.

- Avoid using local tap water while handling your milk and its containers.

- Increase your intake of antioxidants by taking beta-carotene and vitamin E supplements.

Now that we've covered the current recommendations for milk storage and handling, as well as some special situations, next up are the how-to's of feeding your baby with bottles and cups.

6

Feeding Your Baby with Bottles and Cups

If you're like most mothers in Western countries, you have questions about bottle-feeding. At what age should a bottle be introduced? How often should it be given? Who should give it? For some of these questions, there are no definitive answers, but this chapter explains what we do know, and offers suggestions to consider. This chapter also shares strategies that can help you and your caregiver make bottle-feeding more like breastfeeding, so that you can do both in greater harmony. It also covers the introduction of cups, which if you're going back to work when your baby is 7 months or older, may allow you to skip bottles altogether.

When and How to Introduce a Bottle

If you ask friends, relatives, and even health care providers when to introduce a bottle and how often to give it, chances are you will get widely varied and passionate responses. You'll hear stories about babies whose parents waited too long, or didn't give the bottle often enough, and the hardships that occurred when these babies refused the bottle completely. The fact of the matter, though, is that there is very little hard evidence about this. In this way, too, every baby is different.

When to Introduce a Bottle

A story I heard many years ago helped me put the angst that surrounds this issue into perspective. I was helping a breastfeeding mother who was returning to work at the Federal Reserve Bank when her baby was about 6 weeks old. At the same time, she had a co-worker with a new baby about the same age who was also returning to work. The mother I helped did just fine, but the co-worker had challenges. This mother had formula-fed from birth, and when she returned to work at 6 weeks, her baby refused a bottle during his whole first week at daycare.

I was astounded by this story and knew that if she had been a breastfeeding mother, she would have blamed herself. She would have been certain her baby's behavior was all her fault because she had not given the bottle early or often enough, and she would vow to do things differently next time. Obviously, that was not this mother's problem, because her baby had only ever been bottle-fed.

What happened? My assumption was that during maternity leave, this mother and baby had developed a strong bond, and that the baby took one look at the strange caregiver and reacted negatively. It was as if he was thinking, "I don't bottle-feed with anyone but my mother." This story shows that there is much more going on around giving a bottle than most people think. It is not a simple dynamic, and relationships definitely play a role. After hearing this story, I began suggesting that mothers arrange for their babies to spend get-to-know-you time with their caregiver before their first day of work.

In truth, we don't really know the best age to introduce a bottle, although many have passionate opinions. The most common advice is to breastfeed exclusively for the first three to four weeks before introducing a bottle. This strategy gives your baby the practice needed to first master breastfeeding, reducing the chances that he may have a hard time going back to the breast.

Most babies take both breast and bottle just fine. Unfortunately, they aren't born with labels, so you have no way of knowing if your baby can do both early without a problem or if it makes sense to wait a little while. Because it can be gut-wrenching for everyone when a baby refuses the breast, if possible, I think it makes sense to wait the three to four weeks.

How to Introduce a Bottle

Do you really need tips on how to give a bottle? After all, didn't most of us grow up watching babies bottle-feed? Because it's been our cultural norm, we don't usually see ads for bottle-feeding classes. We just assume it's easy to figure out. But if your goal is to bottle-feed in a way that's in harmony with breast-feeding, read on.

Who Should Give the Bottle?

There are two schools of thought on this. One says it's best if the mother avoids giving bottles entirely so that the baby associates bottles with the caregiver and breast with the mother. Those who suggest this approach say it reduces the risk that the baby will grow to prefer the bottle over the breast.

A newer line of thinking says the opposite. Its proponents suggest that it's best for the mother to give the bottle because she knows her baby best and can better gauge the baby's reactions to it (Peterson &

Harmer, 2010). An added benefit to this approach is that the mother is usually more available to do this.

How do you decide? Flip a coin, or go with the approach that makes most sense to you.

Strategies to Prevent Overfeeding

As explained previously, one of the biggest risks associated with the bottle is overfeeding, which is a problem for several reasons. If the milk from the bottle flows really fast, your baby may take a lot more milk than he actually needs while you're at work. This puts pressure on you to provide more pumped milk. Because the volume of milk your baby needs every 24 hours stays relatively stable, overfeeding at work can also lead to less breastfeeding at home, which can throw off your milk production. Consistent overfeeding is also not good for babies, as it promotes unhealthy eating habits, which may increase the risk for overweight or obesity (Li, Magadia, Fein, & Grummer-Strawn, 2012).

The best approach is to try to bottle-feed slowly and mimic breastfeeding dynamics as much as possible. In most cases, each bottle-feeding should take between 15 and 30 minutes. A baby 1 month or older should be satisfied after an average of the 3 to 4 oz. (90-120 mL) he would normally take at the breast. If your baby is younger or is not average and takes more or less at a breastfeeding, aim for your baby's usual intake. If he typically finishes at the breast very quickly, it may make sense for bottle-feeding to take less than 15 to 30 minutes. If feedings are taking longer than 30 minutes or your baby loses interest while bottle-feeding, try a faster-flow nipple.

Keeping bottle-feeding as slow as practical is also the kind thing to do. Science has found more signs of stress among preemies during bottle-feeding than during breastfeeding (Meier, 1988; Meier & Anderson, 1987). A fast, consistent milk flow is harder to control. Imagine trying to drink from a fire hose. If faced with choking or chugging, most babies do their best to chug, but it's not always easy. Thankfully, the following strategies (aka, the "two Ps") can help you make bottle-feeding more manageable for your baby. These strategies would benefit any bottle-fed baby.

Positioning. As with breastfeeding, plan to feed on cue when your baby shows signs of hunger (rooting, hand-to-mouth) but is not yet fussing or upset. The first "P" to help prevent overfeeding is positioning and involves the position of the baby and the bottle. Rather than using the traditional bottle-feeding position, with your baby lying on his back in your arms and the bottle held nearly vertical so that the milk flows fastest, hold your baby more upright and the bottle more horizontally, tipped up just enough so the nipple fills with milk (Figure 10).

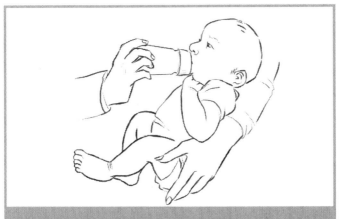

Figure 10. Hold your baby more upright, with the bottle horizontal rather than vertical. ©2014 Anna Mohrbacher. Used with permission.

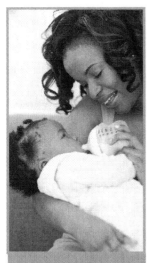

Figure 11. Touch your baby's lips with the nipple and wait until he opens wide before helping him latch on.

With your baby held upright, begin by triggering a wide-open mouth. As with breast-feeding, ideally your baby will take an active role in latching onto the bottle.

- To trigger a wide-open mouth, try tapping your baby's upper lip with the bottle nipple or touching your baby's lips and chin with a gentle, sweeping up-and-down movement (Figure 11).

- When your baby's mouth is open, help him latch onto the nipple so your baby's lips close on the nipple's base rather than its shaft or tip. Latching deeply onto the nipple base will help prevent your baby from developing bad habits with the bottle that can cause breastfeeding problems.

- Check to make sure both your baby's top and bottom lips are flanged out. If they aren't, you can use your fingers to roll them out. If this continues to be an issue, you may want to try a different nipple shape.

If your baby gags when he latches onto the nipple base, this is a sign you either need to use a shorter nipple or the milk is flowing before your baby begins sucking and a slower-flow nipple may be better.

Pacing. The second "P"—pacing—lets you more closely mimic the ebb and flow of the milk during breastfeeding. This way of feeding gives the baby more control over his milk intake.

- When your baby starts feeding from the bottle, build in a pause every few minutes by lowering the end of the bottle so that milk runs out of the nipple. An alternative is to remove the nipple from his mouth, resting the nipple on his lower lip.

- When your baby seems ready to start sucking again, tilt the end of the bottle high enough so that milk partly fills the nipple again or trigger a wide-open mouth so your baby latches again.

- Repeat through the feeding until your baby is done.

Again, expect bottle-feedings to take on average 15 to 30 minutes, and for babies older than 1 month to feel full after about 3 to 4 oz. (90-120 mL). However, let the baby decide when he's done. Just like grownups, babies don't always eat the same amount. Letting your baby set the pace builds healthy eating habits that can last a lifetime.

For step-by-step specifics to share with anyone who feeds your baby, download the Appendix handout, "For the Caregiver of a Breastfed Baby" at: _http://issuu.com/ nancymohrbacher/docs/caregiverbreastfedbabymohrbacher_.

Snacks versus Meals

How much milk to give when you introduce the bottle may sound like a small detail, but it isn't. The reason it looms large, especially during maternity leave, is because if your goal is to exclusively breast-feed, it has a huge impact on how much time each day you spend pumping. Remember, during maternity leave, your top priority is getting in sync with your baby. There will be lots of time for pumping and bottle-feeding later.

If you want your exclusively breastfeeding baby to get a bottle regularly (see next section), think in terms of "snacks" rather than "meals" (Peterson & Harmer, 2010). Specifically, this means giving very small amounts of milk by bottle each day—maybe an ounce (30 mL) each time—rather than a full feeding, and once bottle-feedings are going well, do it less often. This approach has several advantages:

1. It gives your baby practice and familiarity with the bottle (presumably your main goal).

2. It has a minimal impact on normal breast-feeding patterns during a time when frequent feedings are important to establishing your milk production.

3. It minimizes your time spent pumping.

If you're an average pumper, you will likely express the amount of milk you need by just pumping once every other day in the morning about 30 to 60 minutes after your first feeding. You may even need to pump less often than that.

Let's consider the alternative. If instead you give one full bottle-feeding as a substitute for a breast-feeding, for a baby older than 1 month, this would consist of 3 to 4 oz. or 90 to 120 mL of milk. Giving a full feeding could negatively affect your breastfeeding pattern because if your baby takes more from the bottle than from the breast, he may go unusually long before the next feeding. Also, from a practical standpoint, if you're an average pumper, this means you would probably need to pump twice a day to supply this volume of milk. And that doesn't leave any stored milk for other occasions or for your work freezer stash.

As mentioned, few women enjoy pumping. Giving a full bottle-feeding of expressed milk every day requires lots of pumping during maternity leave, which may mean that very quickly you're pumping as often as you will be once you're back at work. Not ideal.

How Often to Give the Bottle

In this area, too, we have no definitive answers, but experience tells us that every baby is different, and there isn't one approach that will work well for all. Keep in mind that there are no guarantees. Some babies fed a bottle each day for their first 3 months decide at that point that they're not going to bottle-feed anymore. Others, who've never had a bottle, take their first bottle at 3 months and never look back. Just like the story earlier in this chapter about the formula-feeding mother whose baby refused a bottle at daycare, giving a bottle regularly does not guarantee that your baby will continue to take one.

That said, you may decide you want to give a bottle regularly because knowing your baby is taking it well gives you peace of mind. If so, what many recommend is that once your baby is taking the bottle well for several days in a row, you can give it less often. Every other day or even every third day is usually often enough to prevent your baby from forgetting how to bottle-feed.

If Baby Resists the Bottle

Many mothers' worst fear is that their baby will refuse a bottle altogether. This is rare, with one study estimating it happens with about 4% of breastfed babies (Kearney & Cronenwett, 1991). This same study also found that about one quarter of babies require some patience and persistence before they take a bottle consistently and well. Don't be discouraged if it takes a little time.

If your baby seems to be resisting the bottle, the most important thing to avoid is allowing the bottle to become a battleground. Continuing to try to give your crying baby a bottle can cause him to develop a negative association with it. Rather than fighting about it, it's much better just to put the bottle down, act like it's no big deal, and try another time.

If your baby has already developed negative associations with the bottle and is upset every time he sees it, you'll need to devote some time to improving his outlook. The key to convincing him that the bottle is really okay is to make all time with the bottle pleasant and positive. Let him play with the bottle on his own with no pressure to take milk. Act like it doesn't matter if he takes it or not. Hold the bottle close to you both while you're playing, smiling, and talking.

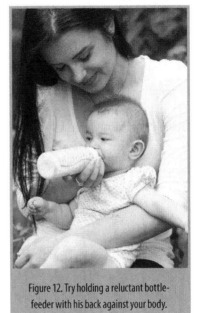

Figure 12. Try holding a reluctant bottle-feeder with his back against your body.

Here are some other tips if your baby resists the bottle.

- Try varying the temperature of the milk. Some babies accept a bottle more easily if the milk is a little warmer or cooler.

- Try offering it at different times of day. Evening is when babies are fussiest and least likely to accept anything new. Try in the morning, when everyone is rested and more cheerful. Pick a time between feedings when your baby is not full and not too hungry.

- Use different feeding positions. Rather than holding your baby in arms in a breastfeeding position, try holding him with his back against yours, or offer the bottle from behind while your baby sits in a car seat or bouncy chair.

Use movement. Some babies will take the bottle better when you're walking or rocking, or even bouncing gently on a yoga ball.

If your baby will take the bottle but just doesn't seem to know what to do with it, try teasing him a little by trying to pull it out. Some babies will respond by sucking it back in.

Nancy Holtzman, RN, IBCLC, CPN, suggests a strategy she calls "Intermittent Bottle by Mom," or IBBM. To do this:

1. Have an ounce (30 mL) or so of freshly expressed milk in a bottle by your feeding spot.

2. Start breastfeeding as usual.

3. After a couple of minutes of breastfeeding, remove the breast and offer the bottle. If your baby takes it, fine. If not, it's no big deal.

4. If your baby didn't take the milk, after another five minutes or so, try the bottle again.

She suggests doing this at three feedings each day. If your baby doesn't take the milk, she suggests putting the bottle in the refrigerator between feedings, rewarming and reusing it until the end of the day, and discarding any remaining milk then.

#1 Tip for Bottle or Breast Refusal

If your baby balks at either breast or bottle, the most important thing is to avoid any fighting or unhappiness. Focus on building positive feelings about it.

If your baby resists the bottle, bring it out only when your baby is calm and happy, and let her play with it. Don't push it. See the IBBM strategy in this chapter.

If your baby begins resisting the breast, focus on creating happy times at the breast with your baby, cuddling, talking, and playing there. Let your baby take a nap with her head resting on the breast. Lean back, and lay your baby tummy down near the breast. Take baths together and build in other times of skin-to-skin contact. Try doing "dream feeds" at the breast, when your baby is in a light sleep (look for eyes moving under eyelids).

Creativity sometimes helps, too. In desperation, one father of a 3-month-old breastfed baby began spooning out some partly defrosted milk and feeding it to his baby like ice cream. His previously unhappy baby, although unwilling to take the bottle, was delighted to eat this new breast-milk "slushie" (Walker, 2011).

Bottle-feeding is a skill that differs from breast-feeding and can take time and practice for some babies to master. Despite what some people say, when babies have trouble taking the bottle, this does not mean they're "being stubborn." And it doesn't make sense to add stress to an already stressful situation by trying to starve them into taking it.

Cup FAQ

It's possible to skip bottles entirely, but nearly every baby eventually learns to use a cup, which is a life-long skill. Many mothers have questions about timing and strategies for transitioning your baby to a cup. The following are some frequently asked questions.

At what age can a baby be fed by cup?

Would you believe that babies can cup-feed from birth? In the West, feeding bottles are common. However, in some parts of the world, bottle-feeding is discouraged. If extra milk is needed, tiny babies sip or lap it from spoons or small, straight-sided cups. Why? In developing countries, water for washing and drinking is not always safe, making it hard to clean bottles and nipples well enough. As a result, mother's milk can become contaminated by the bacteria that grow in the cracks and crevices of a feeding bottle. Even preemies can feed from these straight-sided cups with just a little practice. Canadian pediatrician Jack Newman shows cup-feeding in action in the following free online video: *http://www.breastfeedinginc. ca/content.php?pagename=vid-cupfeed*.

What about cups with lids? Most older babies can manage these on their own at about 7 to 8 months of age. Keep in mind that it may take a couple weeks of practice before your baby takes much milk from the cup.

What do I need to know about cups for older babies?

There are two basic types of commercial cups with lids:

- Cups with built-in straws
- Sippy cups with spouts

In general, cups with straws (Figure 13) are a better long-term choice. Creating a seal on the straw with their lips, sucking on the straw, and then swallowing are appropriate skills for an older baby to master. But you don't need to buy a commercial straw cup. See the next answer for details on strategies for using an open drinking container and a separate straw. Drinking from a straw helps your baby transition more quickly to the types of glasses and cups he will need to use as he grows. Learning to drink from a regular cup and through a straw are skills that babies will use for their entire lives.

In contrast, the mouth movements needed to remove milk from a sippy cup are similar to those used with the bottle. A sippy cup can provide a good short-term transition from bottles, but it is not a necessary step. If a sippy cup is used for years rather than as a short-term transition, one downside is that it teaches tongue thrusting, which can negatively affect your baby's oral development. If sweet liquids such as fruit juice are inside the sippy cup, they can bathe your baby's teeth, which can contribute to tooth decay. For this reason, if you use a sippy cup, consider limiting its contents to water only.

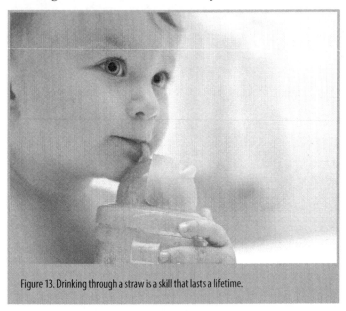

Figure 13. Drinking through a straw is a skill that lasts a lifetime.

What are some tips for getting started with a cup?

When an older baby starts drinking from a cup, put plain water in it while he learns so that you don't have to worry about sticky surfaces or your pumped milk being wasted. Often babies start by turning the cup upside down to see how much spills out and splashing in it. Give your baby a chance to practice with a liquid that is not so precious to you or so likely to make clean-up a challenge.

When you transition your baby to an open cup, or an open cup with a separate straw, a good time to start is when you are sitting next to your baby at mealtimes. While your baby is learning, it may help to shorten the straw by cutting it, as shorter straws require less suction to draw up liquid.

Expect it to take a little time for your baby to go from taking drops from the cup to drinking more. Just like when choosing a bottle, it may help to get a couple of different types and styles of cups to see which your baby prefers.

What should your baby drink from a cup?

For babies between 7 and 12 months, either your milk or water are good choices, as well as clear broths. For babies older than a year, you have more options. Cow's milk from the store is one, which is high in protein and calcium. The American Academy of Pediatrics has long recommended using whole cow's milk until age 2 years, and then switching to 2% milk. Other types of "milks" (more accurately, juices) from beans, grains, and nuts (soy, almond, rice, oat, hemp) are available, too. Soy milk is high in protein. The other "milks" made from plants and nuts are low in protein, but some are calcium fortified.

Plan to keep fruit juice consumption to a minimum. As a natural sugar water, it is missing all of the fruit's healthy fiber. In fact, from a nutritional point of view, fruit juice is not much better than soft drinks. The American Academy of Pediatrics recommends that older babies and toddlers drink no more than 4 oz. (120 mL) of fruit juice per day, as more than this has been linked to health issues (AAP, 2001).

Now that we've covered the basics of cup and bottle-feeding, let's focus on your transition back to work.

7

Resources

Finding Skilled Breastfeeding Help

If you're in need of breastfeeding help, don't wait to find someone. Usually, the sooner you get help, the easier it is to solve your problem. When contacting local breastfeeding specialists, be aware that different credentials reflect different levels of education and training. A variety of initials (CLC, CLE, CBE, CBC, LE, and others) are awarded after attending a brief training course, usually less than one week long. A person with these initials may be able to provide some help but may have limited skills, understanding, and experience.

The credential IBCLC, however, indicates—at the least—a basic competence in the field of lactation. These initials stand for "International Board Certified Lactation Consultant." To receive this credential, a person must pass an all-day certifying exam. To qualify to take that exam, she must first have a combination of formal education, breastfeeding education, and thousands of hours working one-on-one with breastfeeding mothers and babies. There are several ways you can find a local IBCLC.

- Click on the "Find a Lactation Consultant" link on _www.ilca.org_ and enter your ZIP or postal code. ILCA is the International Lactation Consultant Association, the professional association for lactation consultants. Not all international board certified lactation consultants are members.

- Contact your local birthing facility and ask to speak to the breastfeeding specialist. Ask if she can help you or if she knows someone in your community who can.

- Contact your local public-health department and ask if there is any IBCLCs on staff who can help you.

- Contact mother-to-mother breastfeeding support people in your area (see next section) and ask them for suggestions. They may know the best choices in your area.

Another possible source of skilled breastfeeding help is the mother-to-mother support organizations listed in the next section. These experienced breastfeeding mothers work as volunteers to help other mothers. Their skill level can run the gamut from highly skilled to inexperienced. Hopefully, if they can't help you, they'll know someone who can.

Getting the Support You Need

Don't underestimate the importance of ongoing breastfeeding support. What's really great today is that breastfeeding support comes in many forms. Even if you are in a remote location, work odd hours, or lack safe, reliable transportation, you can access the many Facebook groups and online forums that support employed breastfeeding mothers. To get a sense of what's out there and its immense value, see Lara Audelo's book, *The Virtual Breastfeeding Culture: Seeking Mother-to-Mother Support in the Digital Age.*

Mother-to-Mother Breastfeeding Organizations

It's always a plus to have choices, and sometimes there's just no substitute for spending face time with other mothers and babies. Mother-to-mother breast-feeding organizations that offer in-person meetings (as well as online and Facebook support options) are:

- Breastfeeding USA (*www.breastfeedingusa.org*), this rapidly growing nonprofit organization was formed in 2010 with a focus on providing evidence-based information and support in a variety of formats.

- Australian Breastfeeding Association (_www. breastfeeding.asn.au_). This long-standing beacon of breastfeeding support offers a range of services, such as classes, email counseling, a 24-hour Breastfeeding Helpline, online forums, and local support groups.

In the U.K., there are several national breast-feeding support organizations. A list of their links is at: _http://www.nhs.uk/Conditions/pregnancy-and-baby/pages/breastfeeding-help-support.aspx#close_

Another mother-to-mother option in most countries is La Leche League International (_www. llli.org_), the grandmother of breastfeeding support, which has been helping mothers since 1956 and offers in-person meetings, phone, and email help. One way La Leche League differs from other breastfeeding organizations is that it requires its leaders to follow its parenting philosophy, which is consistent with attachment parenting. It does not require those who seek help from La Leche League to follow its philosophy.

Doulas

"Doula" comes from the Greek word for servant, and refers to someone who provides practical and emotional help to women before, during, and after birth. Many doulas also offer breastfeeding help and support.

- DONA International (_www.dona.org_) lists labor-support and postpartum doulas.

- Find a Doula, Australia (_http://www.findadoula. com.au/_) to locale doulas in Australia.

- Doula U.K. (_http://doula.org.uk/_) to locate labor and postpartum/postnatal doulas.

Websites

The internet can be an unreliable place. All breast-feeding websites are definitely not created equal! Here are some that you can trust.

- _Kellymom.com_ is a great site that includes articles on almost every aspect of breastfeeding.

- _NancyMohrbacher.com_ includes a section for employed breastfeeding mothers and many articles on hot topics.

- _BreastfeedingMadeSimple.com_ is the companion site for the book I co-authored with Kathleen Kendall-Tackett, _Breastfeeding Made Simple_. It has many resources for a wide range of breastfeeding concerns and common challenges.

- _WomensHealth.gov/breastfeeding/government-in-action/business-case.html_ Here you can download _The Business Case for Breastfeeding_, which includes materials for mothers, human resources, CEOs, etc. A treasure trove of great resources.

- *Womenshealth.gov/breastfeeding/employer-solutions/index.php* A new U.S. Government website for working and breastfeeding mothers and their employers.

- *BestforBabes.org* offers resources for employed mothers, as well as ways to avoid "booby traps."

- *BreastfeedingPartners.org* Click on the "Work & School" tab to find its *Making It Work Toolkit*, a great resource.

- *Workandpump.com* This site is an oldie but a goodie that is chock full of great info.

- *BreastfeedingUSA.org* offers many helpful articles and a locator for local support.

- *Breastfeedinginc.ca* has many helpful articles and videos by Canadian pediatrician and lactation consultant, Dr. Jack Newman.

- *Isisonline.org.uk* offers evidence-based information for parents and professionals about infant sleep norms.

- *Lowmilksupply.org* was created by two lactation consultants who specialize in milk production issues.

Free Online Videos

Hand Expression:

http://newborns.stanford.edu/Breastfeeding/HandExpression.html

Hands-on Pumping:

http://newborns.stanford.edu/Breastfeeding/MaxProduction.html

Paced Bottle Feeding for the Breastfed Baby:

http://www.youtube.com/watch?v=UH4T70OSzGs&feature=youtube

Reverse Pressure Softening. How to Relieve Engorgement:

http://www.youtube.com/watch?v=2_RD9HNrOJ8&oref=http%3A%2F%2Fwww.youtube.com%2Fwatch%3Fv%3D2_RD9HNrOJ8&has_verified=1

Books

These resources would be great additions to any employed mother's bookshelf.

Audelo, L. (2013). *The virtual breastfeeding culture: Seeking mother-to-mother support in the digital age.* Amarillo, TX Praeclarus Press.

Mohrbacher, N., & Kendall-Tackett, K. (2010). *Breastfeeding made simple: Seven natural laws for nursing mothers, 2nd Ed.* Oakland, CA: New Harbinger Publications.

Mohrbacher, N. (2013). *Breastfeeding solutions: Quick tips for the most common nursing challenges.* Oakland, CA: New Harbinger Publications.

Peterson, A., & Harmer, M. (2010). *Balancing breast and bottle: Reaching your breastfeeding goals.* Amarillo, TX: Hale Publishing.

Rapley, G., & Murkett, T. (2010). *Baby-led weaning: The essential guide to introducing solid foods–and helping your baby to grow up a happy and confident eater.* New York: The Experiment.

Roche-Paull, R. (2010). *Breastfeeding in combat boots: A survival guide to successful breastfeeding while serving in the military.* Amarillo, TX: Hale Publishing.

West, D., & Marasco, L. (2009). *The breastfeeding mothers' guide to making more milk.* New York: McGraw-Hill.

Smartphone App

Here's a basic breastfeeding resource you can download to your Android or iPhone. It covers the 30 most common breastfeeding challenges, and includes the milk-storage guidelines in this book. Use your smartphone to open this link and you're on your way.

Breastfeeding Solutions by Nancy Mohrbacher. (2013). Available for Android and iPhones from Amazon, Google Play, and the App Store. *http://www.nancymohrbacher.com/app-support/*

Breast Pumps to Buy or Rent

Here is the contact information for the three recommended breast-pump brands.

Ameda Breast Pumps

To locate an Ameda rental pump or purchase an
Ameda Purely Yours pump near you, call Ameda
Breastfeeding Products, at 1-866-99AMEDA (1-866-
992-6332), or go online to *www.Ameda.com*.

Hygeia Breast Pumps

To locate a Hygeia rental pump or a Hygeia Enjoye
purchase pump near you, call Hygeia at 1-888-786-
7466 or go online to *www.Hygeiainc.com*.

Medela Breast Pumps

To locate a Medela rental pump or purchase a Medela
Pump In Style or Freestyle pump near you, contact
Medela, Inc., at 1-800-TELLYOU (in the U.S.) or go
online to *www.medela.com*.

Other Products

Hands-Free Pumping Devices

For the latest commercial products that help you
pump hands-free, just Google "hands-free pumping."
Some women make their own. Here are two options:

- This free tutorial uses elastic hair bands: _http://kellymom.com/bf/pumpingmoms/pumping/hands-free-pumping/_

- This one (be sure to click on the pictures) uses rubber bands: _http://www.workandpump.com/handsfree.htm_

Prevent Milk Leakage

To find LilyPadz, the silicone product that applies pressure to the nipples to prevent milk leakage, go online to _www.lilypadz.com_.

Collect Leaked Milk

To find Milkies milk savers, the container you wear to collect milk while your baby breastfeeds, go online to _http://www.mymilkies.com/milksaver_.

References

American Academy of Pediatrics (AAP). (2012). Breastfeeding and the use of human milk. *Pediatrics, 129*(3), e827-e841.

American Academy of Pediatrics. (AAP). (2011). SIDS and other sleep-related infant deaths: expansion of recommendations for a safe infant sleeping environment. *Pediatrics, 128*(5), 1030-1039.

American Academy of Pediatrics. (AAP). (2001). The use and misuse of fruit juice in pediatrics. *Pediatrics, 107*(5), 1210-1213.

Blyton, D. M., Sullivan, C. E., & Edwards, N. (2002). Lactation is associated with an increase in slow-wave sleep in women. *Journal of Sleep Research, 11*(4), 297-303.

Boushey, H., & Glynn, S. J. (2012). There are significant business costs to replacing employees. Retrieved from: http://www.americanprogress.org/wp-content/uploads/2012/11/CostofTurnover.pdf

Brusseau, R. (1998). *Bacterial analysis of refrigerated human milk following infant feeding. Unpublished senior thesis.* Concordia University.

Centers for Disease Control and Prevention. (CDC). (2013). *Unmarried childbearing.* Retrieved from: http://www.cdc.gov/nchs/fastats/unmarry.htm

Centers for Disease Control and Prevention. (CDC). (2012). *Percentage of breastfed U.S. children who are supplemented with infant formula, by birth year.* Retrieved from http://www.cdc.gov/breastfeeding/data/nis_data/

Chatterji, P., & Markowitz, S. (2012). Family leave after childbirth and the mental health of new mothers. *The Journal of Mental Health Policy and Economics, 15*(2), 61-76.

Cohen, R., Lange, L., & Slusser, W. (2002). A description of a male-focused breastfeeding promotion corporate lactation program. *Journal of Human Lactation, 18*(1), 61-65.

Cohen, R., & Mrtek, M. B. (1994). The impact of two corporate lactation programs on the incidence and duration of breast-feeding by employed mothers. *American Journal of Health Promotion, 8*(6), 436-441.

Cohen, R., Mrtek, M. B., & Mrtek, R. G. (1995). Comparison of maternal absenteeism and infant illness rates among breast-feeding and formula-feeding women in two corporations. *American Journal of Health Promotion, 10*(2), 148-153.

Colson, S. D., Meek, J. H., & Hawdon, J. M. (2008). Optimal positions for the release of primitive neonatal reflexes stimulating breastfeeding. *Early Human Development, 84*(7), 441-449.

DaMota, K., Banuelos, J., Goldbronn, J., Vera-Beccera, L. E., & Heinig, M. J. (2012). Maternal request for in-hospital supplementation of healthy breastfed infants among low-income women. *Journal of Human Lactation, 28*(4), 476-482.

Dewey, K. G., & Brown, K. H. (2003). Update on technical issues concerning complementary feeding of young children in developing countries and implications for intervention programs. *Food and Nutrition Bulletin, 24*(1), 5-28.

Doan, T., Gardiner, A., Gay, C. L., & Lee, K. A. (2007). Breast-feeding increases sleep duration of new parents. *Journal of Perinatal and Neonatal Nursing, 21*(3), 200-206.

Dunn, B. F., Zavela, K. J., Cline, A. D., & Cost, P. A. (2004). Breastfeeding practices in Colorado businesses. *Journal of Human Lactation, 20*(2), 170-177.

Geddes, D. T. (2009). The use of ultrasound to identify milk ejection in women: Tips and pitfalls. *International Breastfeeding Journal, 4,* 5.

Goldblum, R. M., Garza, C., Johnson, C. A., Harrist, R., & Nichols, B. L. (1981). Human milk banking I: Effects of container upon immunologic factors in mature milk. *Nutrition Research, 1,* 449-459.

Hale, T. W. (2012). *Medications & Mothers' Milk* (15th Ed.). Amarillo, TX: Hale Publishing.

Hammond, K. A. (1997). Adaptation of the maternal intestine during lactation. *Journal of Mammary Gland Biology and Neoplasia, 2*(3), 243-252.

Heinig, M. J., Nommsen, L. A., Peerson, J. M., Lonnerdal, B., & Dewey, K. G. (1993). Energy and protein intakes of breast-fed and formula-fed infants during the first year of life and their association with growth velocity: the DARLING Study. *American Journal of Clinical Nutrition, 58*(2), 152-161.

Hennart, P., Delogne-Desnoeck, J., Vis, H., & Robyn, C. (1981). Serum levels of prolactin and milk production in women during a lactation period of thirty months. *Clinical Endocrinology (Oxf), 14*(4), 349-353.

Hicks, J. B. (Ed.). (2006). *Hirikani's daughters: Women who scale modern mountains to combine breastfeeding and working.* Schaumburg, Illinois: La Leche League International.

Hill, P. D., Aldag, J. C., Chatterton, R. T., & Zinaman, M. (2005). Comparison of milk output between mothers of preterm and term infants: The first 6 weeks after birth. *Journal of Human Lactation, 21*(1), 22-30.

HRSA. (2008). *The Business Case for Breastfeeding.* Retrieved from: http://www.womenshealth.gov/breastfeeding/govern ment-in-action/business-case-for-breastfeeding/.

Islam, M. M., Peerson, J. M., Ahmed, T., Dewey, K. G., & Brown, K. H. (2006). Effects of varied energy density of complementary foods on breast-milk intakes and total energy consumption by healthy, breastfed Bangladeshi children. *American Journal of Clinical Nutrition, 83*(4), 851-858.

Jones, E., & Hilton, S. (2009). Correctly fitting breast shields are the key to lactation success for pump dependent mothers following preterm delivery. *Journal of Neonatal Nursing, 15*(1), 14-17.

Jones, F., & Tully, M. R. (2011). *Best practices for expressing, storing and handling human milk* (3rd Ed.). Raleigh, NC: Human Milk Banking Association of North America.

Kearney, M. H., & Cronenwett, L. (1991). Breastfeeding and employment. *Journal of Obstetric, Gynecologic & Neonatal Nursing, 20*(6), 471-480.

Kendall-Tackett, K., Cong, Z., & Hale, T. W. (2011). The effect of feeding method on sleep duration, maternal well-being, and postpartum depression. *Clinical Lactation, 2*(2), 22-26.

Kent, J. C. (2007). How breastfeeding works. *Journal of Midwifery & Women's Health, 52*(6), 564-570.

Kent, J. C., Hepworth, A. R., Sherriff, J. L., Cox, D. B., Mitoulas, L. R., & Hartmann, P. E. (2013). Longitudinal changes in breastfeeding patterns from 1 to 6 months of lactation. *Breastfeeding Medicine, 8,* 401-407.

Kent, J. C., Mitoulas, L., Cox, D. B., Owens, R. A., & Hartmann, P. E. (1999). Breast volume and milk production during extended lactation in women. *Experimental Physiology, 84*(2), 435-447.

Kent, J. C., Mitoulas, L. R., Cregan, M. D., Geddes, D. T., Larsson, M., Doherty, D. A., et al. (2008). Importance of vacuum for breast milk expression. *Breastfeeding Medicine, 3*(1), 11-19.

Kent, J. C., Mitoulas, L. R., Cregan, M. D., Ramsay, D. T., Doherty, D. A., & Hartmann, P. E. (2006). Volume and frequency of breastfeedings and fat content of breast milk throughout the day. *Pediatrics, 117*(3), e387-395.

Kent, J. C., Prime, D. K., & Garbin, C. P. (2011). Principles for maintaining or increasing breast milk production. *Journal of Obstetric, Gynecologic, & Neonatal Nursing.* doi: 10.1111/j.1552-6909.2011.01313.x.

Kent, J. C., Ramsay, D. T., Doherty, D., Larsson, M., & Hartmann, P. E. (2003). Response of breasts to different stimulation patterns of an electric breast pump. *Journal of Human Lactation, 19*(2), 179-186.

Kimbro, R. T. (2006). On-the-job moms: Work and breastfeeding initiation and duration for a sample of low-income women. *Maternal & Child Health Journal, 10*(1), 19-26.

Kline, T. S., & Lash, S. R. (1964). The bleeding nipple of pregnancy and postpartum period: A cytologic and histologic study. *Acta Cytologica, 8,* 336-340.

Kramer, M. S., Guo, T., Platt, R. W., Vanilovich, I., Sevkovskaya, Z., Dzikovich, I., et al. (2004). Feeding effects on growth during infancy. *Journal of Pediatrics, 145*(5), 600-605.

Kramer, M. S., & Kakuma, R. (2012). Optimal duration of exclusive breastfeeding *Cochrane Database of Systematic Reviews, Art No. CD003517.*

La Leche League International. (LLLI). (2008). *Storing human milk.* Schaumburg, IL: Author.

Lawrence, R. A., & Lawrence, R. M. (2011). *Breastfeeding: A guide for the medical profession* (7th Ed.). Philadelphia, PA: Elsevier Mosby.

Li, R., Fein, S. B., & Grummer-Strawn, L. M. (2008). Association of breastfeeding intensity and bottle-emptying behaviors at early infancy with infants' risk for excess weight at late infancy. *Pediatrics, 122 Suppl 2,* S77-84.

Li, R., Magadia, J., Fein, S. B., & Grummer-Strawn, L. M. (2012). Risk of bottle-feeding for rapid weight gain during the first year of life. *Archives of Pediatric & Adolescent Medicine, 166*(5), 431-436.

Macknin, M. L., Medendorp, S. V., & Maier, M. C. (1989). Infant sleep and bedtime cereal. *American Journal of Diseases of Children, 143*(9), 1066-1068.

Manohar, A. A., Williamson, M., & Koppikar, G. V. (1997). Effect of storage of colostrum in various containers. *Indian Pediatrics, 34*(4), 293-295.

McGovern, P., Dowd, B., Gjerdingen, D., Dagher, R., Ukestad, L., McCaffrey, D., et al. (2007). Mothers' health and work-related factors at 11 weeks postpartum. *The Annals of Family Medicine, 5*(6), 519-527.

McGovern, P., Dowd, B., Gjerdingen, D., Gross, C. R., Kenney, S., Ukestad, L., et al. (2006). Postpartum health of employed mothers 5 weeks after childbirth. *Annals of Family Medicine, 4*(2), 159-167.

McGovern, P., Dowd, B., Gjerdingen, D., Dagher, R., Ukestad, L., McCaffrey, D., et al. (2007). Mothers' health and work-related factors at 11 weeks postpartum. *Annals of Family Medicine, 5*(6), 519-527.

McKenna, J. J., & McDade, T. (2005). Why babies should never sleep alone: A review of the co-sleeping controversy in relation to SIDS, bedsharing and breast feeding. *Paediatric Respiratory Reviews, 6*(2), 134-152.

Meier, P. (1988). Bottle- and breast-feeding: Effects on transcutaneous oxygen pressure and temperature in preterm infants. *Nursing Research, 37*(1), 36-41.

Meier, P., & Anderson, G. C. (1987). Responses of small preterm infants to bottle- and breast-feeding. *MCN American Journal of Maternal Child Nursing, 12*(2), 97-105.

Meier, P., Motykowski, J. E., & Zuleger, J. L. (2004). Choosing a correctly-fitted breast shield for milk expression. *Medela Messenger, 21*, 8-9.

Mohrbacher, N. (2011). The magic number and long-term milk production. *Clinical Lactation, 2*(1), 15-18.

Mohrbacher, N. (2010). *Breastfeeding answers made simple.* Amarillo, TX: Hale Publishing.

Molbak, K., Gottschau, A., Aaby, P., Hojlyng, N., Ingholt, L., & da Silva, A. P. (1994). Prolonged breast feeding, diarrhoeal disease, and survival of children in Guinea-Bissau. *British Medical Journal, 308*(6941), 1403-1406.

Morton, J., Hall, J. Y., Wong, R. J., Thairu, L., Benitz, W. E., & Rhine, W. D. (2009). Combining hand techniques with electric pumping increases milk production in mothers of preterm infants. *Journal of Perinatology, 29*(11), 757-764.

Morton, J., Wong, R. J., Hall, J. Y., Pang, W. W., Lai, C. T., Lui, J., et al. (2012). Combining hand techniques with electric pumping increases the caloric content of milk in mothers of preterm infants. *Journal of Perinatology, 32*(10), 791-796.

Neville, M. C., Allen, J. C., Archer, P. C., Casey, C. E., Seacat, J., Keller, R. P., et al. (1991). Studies in human lactation: milk volume and nutrient composition during weaning and lactogenesis. *American Journal of Clinical Nutrition, 54*(1), 81-92.

Nichols, M. R., & Roux, G. M. (2004). Maternal perspectives on postpartum return to the workplace. *Journal of Obstetric, Gynecologic, & Neonatal Nursing, 33*(4), 463-471.

Nielsen, S. B., Reilly, J. J., Fewtrell, M. S., Eaton, S., Grinham, J., & Wells, J. C. (2011). Adequacy of milk intake during exclusive breastfeeding: A longitudinal study. *Pediatrics, 128*(4), e907-914.

NWLC. (2012). *The next generation of Title IX: Pregnant and parenting students* [Electronic Version].Retrieved from: http://www.titleix.info/history/history-overview.aspx

Odom, E. C., Li, R., Scanlon, K. S., Perrine, C. G., & Grummer-Strawn, L. (2013). Reasons for earlier than desired cessation of breastfeeding. *Pediatrics, 131*(3), e726-732.

OECD. (2011). *Health at a glance 2011: OECD Indicators: 4.9 Caesarean sections*. Retrieved from: http://www.oecd-ilibrary. org/sites/health_glance-2011-en/04/09/g4-09-01.html?itemId=/content/chapter/health_glance-2011-37-en

Ogbuanu, C., Glover, S., Probst, J., Liu, J., & Hussey, J. (2011). The effect of maternity leave length and time of return to work on breastfeeding. *Pediatrics, 127*(6), e1414-1427.

Ogbuanu, C., Glover, S., Probst, J., Hussey, J., & Liu, J. (2011). Balancing work and family: Effect of employment characteristics on breastfeeding. *Journal of Human Lactation, 27*(3), 225-238; quiz 293-225.

Ortiz, J., McGilligan, K., & Kelly, P. (2004). Duration of breast milk expression among working mothers enrolled in an employer-sponsored lactation program. *Pediatric Nursing, 30*(2), 111-119.

PAHO/WHO. (2001). *Guiding principles for complementary feeding of the breastfed child*. Retrieved from: http://whqlibdoc.who. int/paho/2004/a85622.pdf.

Paxson, C. L., Jr., & Cress, C. C. (1979). Survival of human milk leukocytes. *Journal of Pediatrics, 94*(1), 61-64.

Perrine, C. G., Scanlon, K. S., Li, R., Odom, E., & Grummer-Strawn, L. M. (2012). Baby-Friendly hospital practices and meeting exclusive breastfeeding intention. *Pediatrics, 130*(1), 54-60.

Peterson, A., & Harmer, M. (2010). *Balancing breast & bottle: Reaching your breastfeeding goals*. Amarillo, TX: Hale Publishing.

Pittard, W. B., 3rd, & Bill, K. (1981). Human milk banking. Effect of refrigeration on cellular components. *Clinical Pediatrics, 20*(1), 31-33.

Prime, D. K., Kent, J. C., Hepworth, A. R., Trengove, N. J., & Hartmann, P. E. (2012). Dynamics of milk removal during simultaneous breast expression in women. *Breastfeeding Medicine, 7*(2), 100-106.

Quan, R., Yang, C., Rubinstein, S., Lewiston, N. J., Sunshine, P., Stevenson, D. K., et al. (1992). Effects of microwave radiation on anti-infective factors in human milk. *Pediatrics, 89*(4 Pt 1), 667-669.

Rechtman, D. J., Lee, M. L., & Berg, H. (2006). Effect of environmental conditions on unpasteurized donor human milk. *Breastfeeding Medicine, 1*(1), 24-26.

Roe, B., Whittington, L. A., Fein, S. B., & Teisl, M. F. (1999). Is there competition between breast-feeding and maternal employment? *Demography, 36*(2), 157-171.

SHRM. (2013). *2012 employee benefits research report.* Retrieved from: http://www.shrm.org/research/surveyfindings/articles/pages/2012employeebenefitsresearchreport.aspx

Sievers, E., Oldigs, H. D., Santer, R., & Schaub, J. (2002). Feeding patterns in breast-fed and formula-fed infants. *Annals of Nutrition and Metabolism, 46*(6), 243-248.

Skafida, V. (2012). Juggling work and motherhood: The impact of employment and maternity leave on breastfeeding duration: A survival analysis on Growing Up in Scotland data. *Maternal and Child Health Journal, 16*(2), 519-527.

Slusser, W. M., Lange, L., Dickson, V., Hawkes, C., & Cohen, R. (2004). Breast milk expression in the workplace: A look at frequency and time. *Journal of Human Lactation, 20*(2), 164-169.

Stuebe, A. M., & Rich-Edwards, J. W. (2009). The reset hypothesis: Lactation and maternal metabolism. *American Journal of Perinatology, 26*(1), 81-88.

Stuebe, A. M., Rich-Edwards, J. W., Willett, W. C., Manson, J. E., & Michels, K. B. (2005). Duration of lactation and incidence of type 2 diabetes. *Journal of the American Medical Association, 294*(20), 2601-2610.

Stuebe, A. M., & Schwarz, E. B. (2010). The risks and benefits of infant feeding practices for women and their children. *Journal of Perinatology, 30*(3), 155-162.

Takci, S., Gulmez, D., Yigit, S., Dogan, O., & Hascelik, G. (2013). Container type and bactericidal activity of human milk during refrigerated storage. *Journal of Human Lactation,* *29*(3), 406-411.

Walker, M. (2011). *Breastfeeding and employment.* Amarillo, TX: Hale Publishing.

Walsh, W. (2011). *Single babe breastfeeding: It CAN be done!* Retrieved from: http://www.bestforbabes.org/single-babe-breast feeding-it-can-be-done

Wang, W., Parker, K., & Taylor, P. (2013). *Breadwinner moms.* Washington, DC: Pew Research Center.

West, D., & Marasco, L. (2009). *The breastfeeding mother's guide to making more milk.* New York: McGraw Hill.

Williamson, M. T., & Murti, P. K. (1996). Effects of storage, time, temperature, and composition of containers on biologic components of human milk. *Journal of Human Lactation,* *12*(1), 31-35.

Wilson-Clay, B., & Hoover, K. (2008). *The breastfeeding atlas* (4th Ed.). Manchaca, TX: LactNews Press.

World Health Organization. (WHO). (2010). *Infant and young child feeding.* Retrieved from: http://www.who.int/mediacen tre/factsheets/fs342/en/index.html

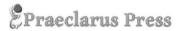

Praeclarus Press

Working and Breastfeeding Made Simple

Nancy Mohrbacher, IBCLC, FILCA

ith its evidence-based insights, *Working
d Breastfeeding Made Simple* takes
e mystery out of pumping and milk
oduction. Written by an international
eastfeeding expert, it puts you in
ntrol of your own experience with
aightforward explanations of how milk
made and what you can do to reach your
vn best level.

hether your maternity leave is long,
ort, or in between, it includes what you
ed to know every step of the way. New
nncepts such as "The Magic Number"
plain how to tailor your daily routine
your body's response. It also includes
mping strategies that can increase your
ilk yields by nearly 50%.

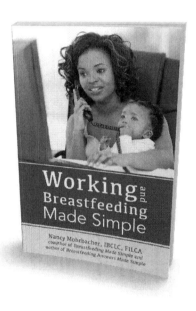

To order a copy, access
http://goo.gl/Kqv6EX, or scan
the QR code below.

Tips from employed mothers provide the
wisdom of hindsight. No matter what
your work setting or whether you stay
close to home or travel regularly, this book
provides the essentials you need to reach
your personal breastfeeding goals.

clarus Press publishes books that change people's
. We want our books to be engaging, grabbing
reader's attention, and beautiful, to nourish
spirits. Smart, but still accessible and practical.
passionate, while reflecting a solid base in
ence. In short, we want them to be excellent.

For a complete list of our books visit
our website, www.praeclaruspress.com,
or scan the QR code on the right.

Made in the USA
Charleston, SC
13 October 2016